DATE DUE

Look
It Up!

Look It Up!

What Patients, Doctors, Nurses, and Pharmacists Need to Know about the Internet and Primary Health Care

PIERRE PLUYE, MD, AND ROLAND GRAD, MD, WITH JULIE BARLOW

McGill-Queen's University Press

Montreal and Kingston • London • Chicago

4/26/18
LN
$29.95

© McGill-Queen's University Press 2017

ISBN 978-0-7735-5136-7 (cloth)
ISBN 978-0-7735-5190-9 (ePDF)
ISBN 978-0-7735-5191-6 (ePUB)

Legal deposit second quarter 2017
Bibliothèque nationale du Québec

Printed in Canada on acid-free paper

McGill-Queen's University Press acknowledges the support of the Canada Council
for the Arts for our publishing program. We also acknowledge the financial support
of the Government of Canada through the Canada Book Fund for our publishing
activities.

LIBRARY AND ARCHIVES CANADA CATALOGUING IN PUBLICATION

Pluye, Pierre, author

Look it up! : what patients, doctors, nurses, and pharmacists need to know about the
Internet and primary health care / Pierre Pluye and Roland Grad with Julie Barlow.
Includes bibliographical references and index.
Issued in print and electronic formats.

ISBN 978-0-7735-5136-7 (hardcover). – ISBN 978-0-7735-5190-9 (ePDF). –
ISBN 978-0-7735-5191-6 (ePUB)

1. Medicine – Computer network resources. 2. Health – Computer
network resources. 3. Internet in medicine. 4. Medical care – Computer
network resources. 5. Medical informatics. I. Barlow, Julie, 1968–, author
II. Grad, Roland, 1960–, author III. Title.

R859.7.I58P58 2017   610.285   C2017-903327-1
                                             C2017-903328-X

This book was typeset by Sandra Friesen in 10.5/13 .5 Minion.

Contents

Foreword

Medical historians estimate that the first time an "average person" had a better than 50:50 chance of being helped, rather than harmed, by consulting a medical clinician was somewhere in the early 1900s. The discovery that germs and cancerous growths caused disease, not bad bile, bad humors, and bad vapors, led to the introduction of antibiotics and chemotherapy agents, handwashing, sterile instruments during surgery, and proper sewage management. For the last 100 years the public has confidently believed that medicine is an asset to public health. We have had faith in the power of health education, disease prevention efforts, diagnosis, prognosis, and treatment to improve lives.

Today, however, many medical and public health scholars, managers, and policy-makers fear that the pendulum has swung the other way. They are concerned that an "average person" may now be more likely to receive harm, rather than benefit, from consulting a clinician.

How can this be?

Simply put, medicine has evolved into a system that is overwhelmed by new technology, diagnostic tests, medicinal drugs, and procedures. As a result, the two greatest risks that patients now face when they consult their doctor are overdiagnosis and overtreatment. Overdiagnosis occurs when someone is given a diagnostic "label" that may lead to harm, from either increased anxiety or unnecessary treatment for a condition that either has no effective treatment or requires no treatment. The harm of overtreatment is more obvious, coming from both known and unexpected adverse outcomes of drugs and procedures. For example, many patients continue to be diagnosed with diabetes on the basis of blood sugar levels for which no treatment, other than diet and exercise, is effective. Many of them receive expensive treatments anyways, then experience adverse effects and increased anxiety, which in turn lead to increased sick time from work and a reduced quality of life.

What can be done to stem the rising tide of overdiagnosis and overtreatment and to address the specter of contemporary medicine becoming a public health hazard? This book takes a huge and necessary step toward stopping and even reversing this trend. Pierre Pluye and Roland Grad have written *Look It Up!* with Julie Barlow for both patients and medical personnel. Drawing on years of their own research, the authors tell real-life stories about clinicians who use electronic knowledge resources to treat patients in a way that is acceptable to both patients and clinicians. One result of clinicians' use of these resources is that it reduces overdiagnosis and overtreatment in medicine. These stories, based on interviews with doctors, nurses, and pharmacists, show that it is possible to make a difference, but that this requires a different type of doctor, nurse, and pharmacist and also a different type of patient.

The clinicians Pluye and Grad describe accept that they can't possibly remember everything. That's why it's so important to be able to accurately "look it up." No one would ever trust a travel agent to rely only their memory to provide detailed information about airlines, flight numbers, flight times, transfer gates, and layover times for a trip from, say, Moose Jaw,

Saskatchewan, to Reykjavik, Iceland. We would expect and even demand that the agent consult the most up-to-date information available on the Internet. In fact, most of us would probably check the information ourselves. Along the same lines, it can no longer be expected that clinicians will rely on their memory alone to handle complex medical problems, and indeed this practice should be unacceptable today. If my 11-year-old daughter were bitten on the finger by a cat and developed a fever and had red streaks spreading up her arm but was allergic to penicillin, I would expect her doctor to check a reliable medical source to determine what antibiotics would be effective in this unusual circumstance before treating her, and not to simply rely on a memory from the distant past.

In this book, Pierre Pluye and Roland Grad explain in clear and understandable language what "shared decision-making" and "evidence-based medicine" mean. It's true that medicine has always been based on evidence, but Pluye and Grad elegantly illustrate how decisions can and should be made on the basis of probability theory and real-world outcomes. Traditional medical education has focused too narrowly on disease pathophysiology. As a result, much medical care treats the individual patient like a complex engineering problem. Through a chain of inductive reasoning that links symptoms and clinical findings to underlying dysfunctions of organs, tissues, and, eventually, cells, clinicians assemble patients into logical puzzles for which they devise diagnostic tests and prescribe treatments aimed at removing the abnormality. In contrast, shared decision-making, as Pluye and Grad show, puts the emphasis on research that directly supports the goal of helping patients to live longer, healthier, and more productive lives.

The stories in this book show how using electronic information helps clinicians determine when a test is likely to be helpful rather than harmful, how it helps them find resolution when disagreements arise, why it is increasingly important to have pharmacists on the health care team, how clinicians and patients can choose the best treatment available, and what specific role patients play in making decisions about their health care. The stories also show the perils and pitfalls of taking unguided trips to the Internet when seeking medical information, the problems that arise in communication between medical providers and their patients, and finally, how to identify that special clinician we all want for ourselves and our loved ones.

The authors have spent much of their careers educating future doctors, nurses, and pharmacists about using electronic information in their practice, helping them to feel good about not knowing everything by focusing on patient-oriented evidence that matters (POEMS) and other information that is valuable to both clinicians and patients. For clinicians, electronic knowledge resources are important because, among other things, trustworthy information will help them to avoid overdiagnosing and overtreating and thereby harming their patients. For patients, electronic knowledge resources can help them live the longest, healthiest, most productive lives they can.

This book takes this same education to the streets. In reading this book, enlightened patients will become more confident about recognizing the uncertainty inherent to medicine, and at the same time they will welcome the clinician who is willing to "look it up." Laypeople reading this book will become those special patients: the other half of the partnership with doctors, pharmacists, or nurses that can change the course of health care and ensure that the health professions are a long-term asset, not a hazard, to public health.

David Slawson, MD
Professor of family medicine, University of Virginia, co-founder of Information Mastery

Acknowledgments

Pierre offers heartfelt thanks to his family, friends, and mentors for their unceasing support, especially Lucie, Mathilde, and Martin, the suns of his life, who genuinely helped to make this book happen. Roland gives special thanks to Corine, his wife, and to his son, Adam. Please share this book with many grandchildren.

We are grateful to all of the nurses, pharmacists, and physicians who generously shared their time and experience. This book is their book. We also thank all of the medical and graduate students, postdoctoral fellows, research professionals, and colleagues who attended our weekly research meetings over the last decade (about 400 two-hour meetings). Their energy, enthusiasm, and ideas always inspired us.

The support of colleagues at the Herzl Family Practice Centre, the Department of Family Medicine at McGill University, and across Quebec, the rest of Canada, and the United States was instrumental in enabling us to write this book. Thank you. Thanks also to the three anonymous reviewers.

Finally, Pierre has been elected fellow of the Canadian Academy of Health Sciences and holds a Senior Investigator Award from the Fonds de recherche du Québec Santé (FRQS). Pierre and Roland have received research grants from the FRQS and the Canadian Institutes of Health Research. We are also grateful to a philanthropic organization (Fondation Lucie et André Chagnon) and to professional organizations (the Canadian Medical Association, the Canadian Pharmacists Association, and the College of Family Physicians of Canada) for their continued support.

Abbreviations

ADHD	attention deficit and hyperactivity disorder
AIDS	acquired immune deficiency syndrome
CPS	*Compendium of Pharmaceuticals and Specialties*
EBM	evidence-based medicine
EMR	electronic medical record
FDA	US Food and Drug Administration
IALS	International Adult Literacy and Life Skills survey
IAM	Information Assessment Method
ICD	International Classification of Diseases
INR	international normalized ratio
NNBI	number needed to benefit from information
OECD	Organisation for Economic Co-operation and Development
POEM	patient oriented evidence that matters
UNESCO	United Nations Educational, Scientific and Cultural Organization
USPSTF	US Preventive Services Task Force
VBAC	vaginal birth after Caesarean

Look
It Up!

Introduction

How does a patient feel when a doctor pulls out a smartphone and starts surfing the Internet in the middle of an appointment? Many are probably puzzled: Aren't doctors supposed to learn everything they need to know in medical school?

Actually, family doctors don't know everything. They couldn't possibly. There's just too much medical information available today for anyone to keep up with the results of all of the latest scientific studies and all of the new and revised clinical practice guidelines for diagnosis, treatment, and prevention. For example, about 22,000 clinical practice guidelines are indexed in MEDLINE (the North American online reference for searching medical publications), and each of those guidelines contains multiple recommendations for a specific health condition.

In and of itself, the profusion of new information isn't a problem. The problem is that family caregivers, doctors, nurses, and pharmacists are not using the abundance of online information that is available to them nearly as much as they could be – or should be – to help patients.

Figuring out exactly why great information is going to waste has been our mission now for over a decade.

Our story actually started back in the 1980s when we began practising family medicine. Searching for clinical information back then was incredibly difficult. There was no Internet, so we had to use bulky reference books and medical journals to find the results of research studies or treatment guidelines for specific diseases and conditions. Printed books were often out of date, and finding recent information in journals was a daunting task. It was practically impossible to find information at the moment we needed it (when we were with a patient and needed to make a diagnosis or a decision). All that would change over the next decade.

We met in 2001 at McGill University's Department of Family Medicine, where we were both doing research (and still are) in the field of information technology in primary care, specifically the use of information and outcomes of information use. At the time, Roland was searching for information on a hand-held computer at the point of care, in his office, while patients were waiting. When it came to new technology, he was what you would call an early adopter among doctors. The medical world was clearly on the verge of an information revolution and the two of us were interested in documenting what was going on. We decided to start collaborating on research to find out how clinicians were using electronic information and how exactly that was helping patients – if indeed it was.

Initially, we were interested in the factors that either prompted clinicians to look it up or discouraged them from doing so and in the impact of point-of-care searches for information on their practice. At that time, there was very little, if any, research about clinicians who used electronic knowledge resources. As a matter of fact, there is still very little research being done today on how primary care clinicians use information content. We were also interested in assessing how patients were being helped when clinicians conducted electronic information searches and used the information they found. This subject seemed like such a fundamental issue to us – the whole point of medicine is to improve people's lives, after all. Typically, however, research studies (outside computer laboratories) assess how frequently clinicians conduct information searches, or they globally assess electronic knowledge resources (with no systematic assessment of the use of specific information).[1] We went on to develop a research method to evaluate information use and subsequent patient outcomes: the Information Assessment Method (IAM).[2] We initially created the online IAM questionnaire for clinicians, but we have subsequently developed versions for consumers, managers, and parents, and they are all available on our website (www.mcgill.ca/iam). The IAM questionnaire was developed through publicly funded research and we have done a number of studies to document its validity.[3]

The IAM Internet-based questionnaire for clinicians asks them to rate the relevance, cognitive impact, intended use, and expected patient health benefits of information they retrieve or receive. For example, the questionnaire simply asks physicians and pharmacists to rate brief pieces of electronic information they receive. Most clinicians today receive email alerts of clinical information on a regular basis from commercial, professional, or governmental sources. This is true across the planet, although as far as we know the integration of professionally pre-appraised, non-commercial email alerts into clinicians' continuing education programs is only happening in Brazil, Canada, and the United States. Examples of these alerts are daily POEMs (bottom-line synopses of new research studies that are produced in the United States and emailed to members of the Canadian Medical Association) and weekly "Highlights" (summaries of research results and guidelines from an electronic textbook produced by the Canadian Pharmacists Association and emailed to their members and to members of the College of Family Physicians of Canada).

If Canadian pharmacists and physicians rate the information they receive using the IAM, they earn continuing education credits (pharmacists and physicians are obligated to do a certain amount of continuing education to maintain their practice competency). The IAM was an immediate success when it was introduced in 2005, and it continues to be successful. Between 20 January and 31 December 2010, we received 31,429 Highlight ratings from 5,346 family physician participants. For 90% of these rated Highlights, the physicians indicated the information they retrieved was relevant to at least one of their patients. For 41% of the rated Highlights, physicians expected at least one patient to benefit if they implemented the recommendation, whether that meant avoiding an unnecessary treatment, proceeding with a preventive intervention, or improving a patient's health.[4] To date, we have collected more than two million responses to our questionnaire from more than 15,000 pharmacists and physicians involved in Highlight and POEM continuing education programs. Our work is part of an emerging research area called big data, involving huge data sets that researchers use to identify trends and relationships between variables.[5]

However, although the IAM allows us to measure clinicians' intention to use the electronic information they receive and the benefits they expect to get from this use, it does not tell us anything about which clinical situations they use the information in, or why or how they use it. More specifically, it does not tell us whether the information actually leads to positive patient outcomes. In other words, it does not tell us whether information searches actually help patients. So, starting in 2004, we added another element to our research. Our team began to conduct interviews with volunteers from among our IAM questionnaire users. We sat down with them in person or talked to them by phone, and we asked them to describe exactly how they had used the information they had rated to help a specific patient. We wanted to know what information use meant in practice and what the consequences were for the patient and their family. Study participants were family medicine residents, family physicians, primary care nurse practitioners, and community pharmacists. Using the information they had rated as our starting point, we asked them to describe the entire story of finding and applying the information in specific cases. The stories in this book are drawn from over a decade of these interviews. Most of the interviews were conducted by a qualified medical anthropologist. We structured the questions using a well-known and well-accepted process theory in information sciences called the acquisition-cognition-application model.[6] This model explains how information is valuable from a user perspective. It allows us to systematically describe how thinking and behaviour unfold when clinicians (or anyone else) look for information to apply to a specific goal. In our research studies, the model formalized how clinicians assimilated and applied electronic information: first they searched electronic knowledge resources for clinical information to fulfill a specific objective (acquisition), then they integrated relevant information with their previous knowledge (cognition), and then they applied it to a particular patient's situation (application). To make the interviews even more specific, we analyzed participants' answers according to four levels of outcomes.[7] In technical terms, we documented the situational relevance of the retrieved information content, whether the information had positive cognitive impact, whether it was used in the management of a patient, and, whether it led to a patient health benefit. These elements correspond roughly to the process of skimming through hits in an Internet search, finding something relevant, reading it, processing it, making a decision about whether to use it or not, and describing what came of that information. We then merged the quantitative data (IAM ratings) and qualitative data (interviews and documents such as log reports and information content) into clinical vignettes (see http://iamclinical vignettes.mcgill.ca and http://iamclinicalvignettes2.mcgill.ca). Each vignette serves as a story that explains how a clinician used the information: why they looked for it, how they made sense of it, how they applied it, and what the ultimate outcome was. The stories also include patients and their relatives, who often played a role in the process, collaborating with, questioning, or even challenging clinicians at different stages. In the world of health and social sciences, this is called mixed methods research.[8] We combined the collection and analysis of quantitative data (thousands of responses to the IAM questionnaire were analyzed using statistics) with the collection and analysis of qualitative data (interviews and documents were interpreted by researchers using themes derived from a theoretical model and suggested by the interviewees). Up to now, only mixed methods research studies like the ones we conducted have had the potential to establish a systematic chain of evidence between specific information content retrieved in routine practice and reported benefits for a particular patient. In the stories that resulted from our research we changed the names and circumstances of patients, family caregivers, nurses, pharmacists, and physicians to preserve anonymity (in accordance with the ethics guidelines of our university), but the stories themselves are real.

It should be noted that our stories come only from primary care clinicians, and the ones who participated are more likely to search online for information than the average clinician. If we wanted to be able to generalize our results to the entire population of clinicians in the classic statistical manner, we would have to conduct our research with large, random samples from all disciplines. But it would be impossible for us to conduct this type of study for the simple reason that not all clinicians use electronic knowledge resources in the same way. Given the diversity of resources available, the ease with which they can be accessed, and the diversity of information needs and uses, it would be impossible to track and assess all information searches from such samples. Besides, producing results that are statistically generalizable is not really our purpose. We are not working in a laboratory to replicate a controlled experiment on one chemical substance, nor are we working in a field of traditional scientific research such as physics.

We conduct exploratory research on a variety of everyday primary care practices in the field of knowledge translation, which is defined as "a process including dissemination and application of knowledge to improve health services and health."[9] The purpose of our research is to determine the meaning of information use (and expected benefits for patients) from a clinician's perspective, something that has never been done before, and to see whether, and in what ways, patients can benefit from clinicians' use of specific medical information derived from electronic knowledge resources.

Information studies suggest there are six types of situations where clinicians look for information – or don't. A typical situation is where clinicians don't look for information when they need it because they are too busy. There is also the situation where clinicians simply don't think of looking something up, since they don't know what they don't know (this is called unknown information needs). In addition, there is the situation where there is no answer to a clinician's question in the medical literature. In another situation, clinicians aren't able to find the answer that is available or disagree with the answer they find, or they feel it would be harmful to their patient. A few computer-laboratory studies suggest there is a rare situation where clinicians find a wrong answer to a clinical question. Finally, there is the situation where a clinician faces a clinical question, looks it up, finds the right answer, and uses it for a specific patient who may benefit from the information.

The stories in this book involve clinicians in this final situation: doctors, nurses, and pharmacists who turned to an electronic information source to find an answer, or answers, to a clinical question; felt the information they found had a positive impact on them personally, in terms of their own lifelong learning; used the information for a particular patient; and found that the information sometimes benefited the health of this patient. Overall, we interviewed 85 clinicians (doctors, nurses, and pharmacists) and collected 402 clinical stories where the clinician used the information she/he found for a particular patient.[10]

Our method (IAM) and study results (descriptive) show that patients can frequently benefit from information delivered by or retrieved from electronic knowledge resources (for more information, please see our publications list at www.mcgill.ca/iam). We also developed a score for illustrating how beneficial information searches might actually be. We call this the number needed to benefit from information (NNBI). According to our studies, the NNBI (the number of patients for whom clinical information has to be retrieved in order for one patient to benefit) varies from six to 14. In one of our studies, 39 practising family physicians from across Canada rated 1,193 searches for information over an average of 86 days; 715 of the searches were done for a patient.[11] In 365 of these searches, physicians reported some information use, which we documented through interviews. In 53 of the searches, participants described how the use of retrieved information had led to at least one patient health benefit. There were 715 patients for whom information was found and 53 of these searches led to a patient benefit. This works out to a ratio of 13.5 searches for one patient benefit (715/53 = 13.5), which we rounded to "14 for 1" as there are no half-patients.

What's more, our studies suggest that while the NNBI might be up to 14 for family medicine residents and family physicians, it may be around six for primary care nurse practitioners and pharmacists.[12] These numbers provide the groundwork for useful plausible hypotheses for further research. We also have reason to believe that the actual NNBIs might be lower (i.e., it might take fewer information searches to get information-related benefits) in the general population of practitioners. This is because the clinicians who volunteered to participate in our study were probably higher users of electronic knowledge resources than the general population of practitioners.

The NNBI is a novel idea that needs to be remeasured in future studies, using different electronic knowledge resources and innovative experimental methods. Still, what we discovered should encourage clinicians to systematically search for clinical information when they feel they need it. The high likelihood of positive outcomes from these searches should also give patients more incentive to seek information on their own (or with relatives and friends when necessary) or to ask clinicians and librarians to look for trustworthy information on their behalf.

In writing this book, our objective was to explain what our research findings mean in everyday life, using the stories we have collected. It was also to dig deeper and explain how and why clinicians use – or don't use – information from electronic knowledge resources. Clinicians' individual inclinations and information needs, of course, play a large part in their decisions to search for information in these resources, but this is not the whole story. Clinicians' behaviour with respect to electronic knowledge resources has also been shaped by the evolution of the practice of medicine, and that's a part of the story we also wanted to tell.

The story of this book really started some 25 years ago, before the use of the Internet became widespread, at McMaster University in Hamilton, Ontario. A group of doctors there developed a revolutionary concept they called evidence-based medicine. Their idea was simple enough: they wanted to encourage doctors to make the fullest possible use of scientific research results when treating patients. It was a great idea but an impossible one to apply, mostly because doctors had to travel to academic libraries, which were often some distance away, to find the latest research on diseases or treatments, and they could not read and appraise all scientific publications relevant to their patients in a timely manner.

Today, trustworthy medical information is available 24/7, from almost anywhere, for patients, family caregivers, and all health care professionals; specifically, doctors, nurses, and pharmacists learn about evidence-based medicine as part of their training. The fact that medical information is easily available to everyone not only allows patients to participate more in their own treatment through the widely accepted practice of shared decision-making, it also enables clinicians to find answers, reduce uncertainties, check for alternative treatment options for patients, and do much more, in just minutes. Electronic knowledge resources provide information (including updated syntheses of critically appraised research results) that is making it possible to cut medical costs by avoiding unnecessary tests or treatments.

However, as we discovered, technology has changed faster than attitudes. While reliable electronic knowledge resources have been developed at an amazing speed, neither clinicians nor patients are using these resources as much as they could. Many patients still expect medical professionals to have all the answers, so when they see their clinician looking for online information during a consultation they don't consider it a good thing. Many doctors, meanwhile, are aware of their patients' doubts and avoid looking online in their patients' presence out of fear that doing so will make them look less competent. As we describe later, research shows that family physicians do not search for information (when they should) about half of the time.

What's going on? One problem is how doctors have been trained to see themselves: as experts who are supposed to know it all. In this age of easily accessible online information, most doctors, nurses, and pharmacists think differently about how they work. With so much information available, they have to start looking at what they do in their daily practice not as holding a whole bunch of information in their heads but as part of a process of lifelong learning. All of the information they need is there – electronic information resources can be seen as an unlimited external memory. The information just has to be used for the right patient at the right time. As these stories show, both clinicians and patients have a role to play in making sure information gets found and then used in a timely manner.

We feel that it's important from the outset to clarify the relationship between this book and the evidence-based medicine (EBM) movement as a whole, in particular because a number of clinicians and researchers have criticized, and continue to criticize, EBM. Their view is that EBM devalues clinical experience and intuition in favour of hard science.

That perception, though misguided, is understandable. When EBM was first developed at McMaster University in the early 1990s, the founders of the movement called it scientific medicine. That sparked a belief among some members of the medical community that EBM's founders were pushing clinicians to diagnose and treat patients *entirely* on the basis of scientific evidence – and more specifically on the basis of the results of randomized controlled trials (hereafter called trials). Trials typically involve two groups, with eligible participants randomly assigned to each group. In one group the participants receive an experimental intervention (e.g., a potentially beneficial medication), and in the other group, called the control group, the participants receive standard care or no intervention (e.g., a placebo). The results of the two groups are then compared.

To address this perception – and to dispel the belief that the movement proposed blindly applying results from trials – the founders renamed it evidence-based medicine. From the outset, the objective of EBM was not to do away with clinical judgment. The movement was born out of the realization that while physicians commonly used their experience in diagnosing and treating, they rarely used research results. The founders of EBM wanted clinicians to combine experience and research. As they explained, "the practice of evidence-based medicine means integrating individual clinical expertise with the best available external clinical evidence from systematic research."[13] Twenty years later, in a poignant essay, Iona Heath (an English physician, writer, and former president of the Royal College of General Practitioners) reminded us that research results (evidence) come from studies of populations.[14] Citing a paper

BOX 1 THE RENEWED EVIDENCE-BASED MEDICINE FRAMEWORK.

REAL EVIDENCE BASED MEDICINE
- Makes the ethical care of the patient its top priority
- Demands individualised evidence in a format that clinicians and patients can understand
- Is characterised by expert judgment rather than mechanical rule following
- Shares decisions with patients through meaningful conversations
- Builds on a strong clinician-patient relationship and the human aspects of care
- Applies these principles at community level for evidence-based public health

ACTIONS TO DELIVER REAL EVIDENCE BASED MEDICINE
- Patients must demand better evidence, better presented, better explained, and applied in a more personalised way
- Clinical training must go beyond searching and critical appraisal to hone expert judgment and shared decision making skills
- Producers of evidence summaries, clinical guidelines, and decision support tools must take account of who will use them, for what purposes, and under what constraints
- Publishers must demand that studies meet usability standards as well as methodological ones
- Policy makers must resist the instrumental generation and use of "evidence" by vested interests
- Independent funders must increasingly shape the production, synthesis, and dissemination of high quality clinical and public health evidence
- The research agenda must become broader and more interdisciplinary, embracing the experience of illness, the psychology of evidence interpretation, the negotiation and sharing of evidence by clinicians and patients, and how to prevent harm from overdiagnosis

Reproduced, with permission from BMJ Publishing Group Ltd., from T. Greenhalgh, J. Howick, and N. Maskrey, "Evidence-Based Medicine: A Movement in Crisis?" *British Medical Journal* 348 (2014): g3725.

by Alvin Feinstein on clinical judgment, she added that trial-based evidence can only inform us about probabilities; it can never predict what will happen to an individual because trials (and all quantitative studies) "are deliberately aimed at showing average efficacy in a diseased group rather than optimum management for an individual patient." These issues are being addressed by the development of genetic personalized medicine, the person-centred medicine movement (defined as the "articulation of science and humanism to enhance personalized understanding of illness and positive health, clinical communication, and respect for the dignity and responsibility of every person" by the *International Journal of Person Centered Medicine*), and the renewal of EBM.[15]

The idea of what constitutes EBM has evolved. Those who teach and write about EBM today (ourselves included) promote a much broader definition of evidence than what the movement's early leaders had in mind. But the efforts to redefine the traditional conception of EBM have met with resistance both from those who oppose the principle and those who believe EBM should only include evidence from trials. In 2016, Pierre, along with 80 other senior academics from 11 countries around the world, signed a letter to the editors of the highly respected *British Medical Journal* asking them to reconsider their longstanding policy of refusing to publish studies that used qualitative and mixed methods research.[16] This journal is a resource for both primary care clinicians and researchers, and that letter went on to be one of the most frequently cited publications in social media that the journal has ever published. In short, the debate about what EBM is, and what place it should have in medical practice and research, is still a hot one.

Our research and this book are consistent with the renewed version of EBM (box 1) proposed by Professor Trish Greenhalgh (a practising family physician and an internationally recognized academic leader in primary health care research) and colleagues.[17]

Randomized controlled trials actually constitute a small fraction of the evidence used by the clinicians in our stories. The nurses, pharmacists, and physicians in our stories obtain and apply evidence from their patients (including relatives) and their clinical experience, as well as colleagues' advice, experts' recommendations, organizational routines and policies, and research results. In line with the renewed EBM that we espouse, the clinicians in our stories use at least three types of sources of evidence (patient, clinician, and organization) and the best available information (codified knowledge) from multiple forms of research evidence (results from theoretical research, methodological research, and empirical qualitative, quantitative, and mixed methods research) when providing health education and preventing, diagnosing, and treating health conditions and problems.

Our stories also illustrate the growing movements in clinical practice that are, in turn, broadening the scope of evidence that clinicians use. At the individual level, there are movements promoting patient engagement in health care and shared decision-making. At the level of society as a whole, movements are promoting the participation of patient as partners in the management of health organizations and research. For example, Pierre leads the method development component of a state-level patient-oriented research unit that promotes active patient participation (co-decision-making and co-construction of scientific knowledge) in planning and conducting primary care research. In line with these movements, we conceive information use ("look it up") as a way for knowledge from both the health system (information found by doctors, nurses, and pharmacists) and the consumer system (information found by patients directly and through their social networks) to be accessed, merged, and applied. Luhmann, a famous contemporary sociologist, explains this as the interpenetration of social systems centred on communicative action.[18]

In short, the 33 stories in this book illustrate many facets of renewed EBM as it is applied in everyday practice. In seven of these stories, clinicians used the results of randomized controlled trials as their main source of evidence, which they interpreted in the context of the clinical situation they were facing. In 11 stories, clinicians used other forms of quantitative research evidence, such as the results of observational studies. Qualitative research findings were used in three stories; a medical case report was used in one; and health policy was used in another. All 33 stories show how clinicians interpret and integrate research-, expert-, and policy-based evidence found in high-quality electronic knowledge resources with patient evidence (mixing contingencies and free will) they gleaned from conversations with patients and families.

It may come as a surprise to many readers, but trials are not the most common type of research in medicine today. MEDLINE contains about 22.3 million records; about 10.1 million of these (or 45%) report the results of qualitative, quantitative, or mixed methods research studies whereas only 421,000 (or 2%) are records for randomized controlled trials. Trials measure the effectiveness of simple prevention and treatment interventions, for instance, but it may be neither feasible nor ethical to carry out this type of study in many situations.[19] Other types of research designs may be more appropriate for studying certain issues. For example, qualitative research is good for exploring patients' experience, and observational quantitative research studies are good for measuring the importance of a problem. For an emerging health problem that has not yet been explained, its description starts with a case report. A good example of this would be the first observed cases in the 1970s of the infection that later came to be known as HIV. Another consideration is that much preliminary research is needed before a randomized controlled trial can be designed. In sum, "there is no trial evidence" does not mean "there is no appropriate research evidence."

We believe the Internet will help make doctor visits – or consultations with a pharmacist or nurse – better in almost every way in the future. To contribute to this future, we wrote this book with a large audience in mind, including patients, family caregivers, nurses, pharmacists, and physicians, and we adopted a health promotion approach as we were crafting the manuscript. After you read the patient stories in this book, which we selected from the hundreds we collected in our research and from the stories arising from our own experience, we are confident you will know what to do to make this future happen.

Proviso

Knowledge in health sciences and medicine is constantly evolving, and best practices may have changed since we wrote this book. Thus, we ask the reader to critically examine our clinical stories and look or ask for updated knowledge when it seems necessary.

Chapter 1

A New Way of Diagnosing

Roland will never forget the day Anne, one of his patients, bluntly asked him, "Why would I want to see a doctor who has to look things up on the Internet?"

Anne had sprained her ankle. Traditionally doctors send patients with sprained ankles to a clinic or the hospital to get an X-ray, just to be sure nothing is broken, then refer them to an orthopaedic specialist. Roland knew Anne wouldn't have a problem with this. A well-off, middle-aged woman, she understood how the medical system worked and was used to consulting specialists. She had the time and the means to get as much care and as many second opinions as she felt she needed.

Yet Roland hesitated. He was pretty sure Anne hadn't broken her ankle. Even so, he wanted to be really sure before sending her home to put ice on it. Roland knew it would only take him a minute or so to check. He pulled out his smartphone.

Anne squirmed and raised her eyebrows sceptically. This was the first time she had seen a doctor looking up information on the Internet right in front of her – and on a smartphone, of all things.

But her discomfort didn't last long. In a matter of seconds Roland found what he needed on one of the websites he regularly consulted: a diagram of two feet with six questions underneath them, called simply the Ottawa Ankle Rules. The Ankle Rules were developed by researchers at the University of Ottawa to help emergency doctors quickly decide which patients with ankle injuries should have X-rays and which ones shouldn't.

Following the guidelines of the Ankle Rules, Roland asked Anne exactly where her pain was. Could she bear weight on the ankle? When she answered that she could, Roland knew she didn't need an X-ray.

Anne was a regular patient, and Roland knew she was the type to say exactly what was on her mind. When she asked why a doctor would need to look up medical information on his smartphone, she was expressing doubts that a lot of Roland's patients had but were too shy to ask about.

As more and more doctors pull out smartphones and tablets before prescribing a treatment, or even before diagnosing a patient's problems, lots of people, like Anne, will wonder just what the world has come to. Do doctors really need to go onto the web to figure out how to diagnose things these days? Don't they learn everything they need to know in medical school?

Well, yes and no. If Anne had come to Roland with a sprained ankle even a decade ago, he would have made an educated guess about whether or not she needed an X-ray. He would probably have erred on the side of caution and sent her for an X-ray just in case.

Today, thanks to his hand-held device, Roland has access, in less than a minute, to reliable websites with up-to-date medical information. By using this device, he can provide better, more thorough answers to his patients' questions, save them time and unnecessary medical treatments, or even find information about treatments he might not have known about.

So it's a good thing clinicians can look things up quickly on Internet. And it's especially good for family physicians.

What's so special about family doctors? Family physicians are often the first clinicians people see when they have a problem. That means family physicians see a wider variety of problems than any other kind of medical professional. Take ankle sprains. Orthopaedic surgeons and emergency medicine specialists see them every day. (In fact, as Roland later learned, orthopaedic surgeons use the Ottawa Ankle Rules so often they don't need to look them up.)

But family physicians like Roland, who work in offices, don't see sprained ankles that frequently. So, naturally, family doctors are somewhat less familiar with the latest diagnostic tools for ankle injuries – or any other specific disease, illness, or injury, for that matter – and need to "look it up" to get the latest information.

So it's a good thing doctors have the Internet, isn't it?

There are lots of people, like Anne, who react instinctively and don't consider it a good thing at all. For many patients, it is disturbing to see a health professional turn to the Internet for information right in front of their eyes. Doctors who "look it up" can come across as doctors who don't know what they are doing. Instead of thinking, "Gee, it's great that my doctor wants to know the most up-to-date information to answer my questions," patients like Anne think, "What kind of doctor needs to Google things?"

A few years ago, medical researchers published the results of a study called "Must We Appear to Be All-Knowing?" in the journal *Canadian Family Physician*.[1] They documented patient attitudes about doctors who consulted electronic knowledge resources. Almost two out of five patients reported that watching a doctor search the Internet during a consultation decreased their confidence. Worse, they found that for almost one-third of patients, watching a doctor search the Internet actually made them feel they were getting a lower quality of care.

What explains this negative perception? The first factor is plain old habit. When people go to the doctor, they expect to get an answer. That's the way we've traditionally been taught to think about medicine.

In fact, many patients' expectations were shaped by the world before smartphones, the Internet, and high-speed computers. Back then – and we're only talking about two decades ago – doctors didn't know more, or remember more, than they do now. They still would have benefited from looking things up; they just couldn't do it as easily. If a doctor wanted specific information about a condition, he or she had to go to a library, flip through a card index, and read entire scientific papers. What patient would have liked being told by a doctor, "I'll get back to you next week when I've had a chance to look into it"?

In other words, doctors didn't look things up for the simple reason that it took too long. So doctors made their best guess. They were usually right, but not always.

Today, doctors and patients live in a different world. As we said earlier, it's not that doctors know less than they used to. It's that they now have the ability to continually add to their body of knowledge, because they can get information from an electronic database in seconds. They can't possibly know every bit of medical information that is available at any given time – especially as research creates new information every day.

Older patients are the most likely to look with a sceptical eye at doctors searching the Internet. As one physician explained during an interview with Pierre, "I think you have to be careful when you have an older patient who doesn't understand technology. They may really wonder, 'What's the doctor doing fiddling around with this computer?' and you have to be careful. You can't become all absorbed in your little machine and lose sight of the patient because you will break the relationship and you might break your patient's confidence."

Even young, technologically savvy patients may have doubts about doctors surfing the web in front of them. It's not that these patients distrust their doctors. Instead, they somewhat distrust the Internet. They know that not all information on the Internet is trustworthy – in fact, far from it.

Another problem is that some patients have unrealistic expectations about doctors. Even if most patients know that no one can know everything, for some reason they think that doctors should. Watching a doctor look for information brings out their worst fear: that there is no answer to their problem.

Patients aren't the only ones who have qualms about using the Internet. In their pioneering information studies in primary care, John Ely (professor emeritus of family medicine, University of Iowa Carver College of Medicine) and colleagues found that about half the time, family physicians who know they need information decide not to search for it.[2] A recent systematic review of research studies confirmed this finding: across 11 studies, 7,012 clinical questions were elicited through short interviews with clinicians (mostly primary care physicians and nurses) after each patient visit. On average, clinicians reported one question every two patients, but they did not look for information regarding half of their questions. Worse still, the authors of the review noted that "this picture has been fairly stable over time despite the broad availability of online evidence resources that can answer these questions."[3] Thus, our book addresses an ongoing issue.

Why don't clinicians seek answers to their questions? Physicians say the main reason is lack of time. In Canada, for instance, family physicians are usually paid per patient encounter, so the more patients they see, the more money they make. Naturally, in this system, some feel that if they slow down appointments to spend time searching for information, they will "lose" money. And the problem is not just the time they spend searching. It's also the time they spend explaining the information they find to patients.

Money is not the only thing that discourages physicians from consulting electronic knowledge resources. Patients' attitudes

– or what doctors perceive as patients' attitudes – also discourage doctors from doing information searches during consultations. It's a classic case of reality versus perception. From a professional viewpoint – that is, from the viewpoint of clinicians – if a doctor is looking for information it's considered a sign that he or she has a high-quality practice. From a patient's perspective, however, information searches can look like a sign of a low-quality practice.

This, as we'll see, creates a kind of vicious circle where good information literally goes to waste. Some clinicians, fearing a patient will react negatively to seeing them look up information on a hand-held device, choose to leave the consultation room to do searches. But others simply avoid doing information searches altogether, even when they know they should.

The other problem is the way doctors see themselves. Many doctors believe that they should know everything, or at least everything they need to know to do their job. After all, doctors get into medical school largely because they *can* keep a lot of information in their heads. Many doctors leave medical school convinced they should know all the answers by heart.

That attitude might have made sense in an age before the advent of electronic databases, when doctors really didn't have a choice but to try to keep as much information in their heads as possible. But today, thanks to electronic knowledge resources, there is more medical information available than ever: guidelines, syntheses and synopses of clinical research, decision support systems (expert systems containing decision rules based on mathematical algorithms), electronic journals, textbooks, and medical websites. With the simple stroke of a touch screen, doctors can now find information that wasn't accessible even 15 years ago. There is so much information available today – information that can improve, or maybe even save, lives – that doctors simply can't know it all.

This is particularly true for family doctors. Pierre had an eye-opening experience with an ophthalmologist that reminded him why the work of family physicians is so different than that of other medical specialists. During a regular eye checkup, Pierre's optometrist thought he saw early signs of glaucoma, so he sent Pierre to a glaucoma clinic to have it checked out. Pierre spent the whole morning at the clinic. The experience made him feel like the tramp in Charlie Chaplin's movie *Modern Times*: Pierre felt like he was trapped inside a machine that was slowly "processing" him.

When he arrived at the clinic, Pierre went to the receptionist to get a number. Then, when his number was called, he saw Technician Number One, who told him, "Look here and click the button when you see the spot." He looked, clicked, and returned to his seat in the waiting room until his number was called again. Then he saw Technician Number Two, who told him to look at a screen and tell him what he saw. He looked, answered, and then went back to his seat again.

The next time he was called, he finally saw the ophthalmologist. The specialist reported mechanically: "Tests normal. Your optometrist made an error. You don't have glaucoma. Call back in four years to schedule a routine checkup. You probably don't need it but it's better to be sure. Goodbye."

The whole discussion took three minutes.

At the ophthalmology clinic, Pierre felt like he had been processed through a series of mechanical procedures and impersonal exchanges. In fact, there was nothing wrong with the impersonal service. Pierre had no particular need to develop relationships with any of the medical professionals he encountered there – nor they with him. Specialists and technicians in ophthalmology see cases of glaucoma many times a day and they know how to diagnose it quickly and efficiently. That's exactly what the team at this clinic did.

In short, specialists see the same specific problems over and over, every day. So they become extremely knowledgeable about the few guidelines governing their particular fields of practice. By drawing on their own knowledge and experience, they can

make diagnoses quickly, usually without having to look anything up.

The work of family doctors is exactly the opposite. In contrast to other specialists, primary care clinicians usually
establish long-term relationships with patients and their families and are the main point of entry to the medical system. They
are also usually responsible for the continuity, comprehensive-
ness, and coordination of health care services outside hospitals.
Both patients and physicians say they value the close relationship they develop over time.[4]

Among different kinds of doctors, family physicians encounter the widest range of health conditions in their day-to-day
work. Specialists are trained to use algorithms, which are step-
by-step procedures, to make diagnoses. Family doctors could
not possibly learn, let alone retain, all the algorithms doctors
use to diagnose every problem they encounter.

To get an idea of how many different problems family doctors treat, consider this list of the top 14 reasons people consult
a family doctor: high blood pressure; vaccination; infection like
influenza, sinusitis, or pharyngitis; depression; diabetes; lipid
disorders (like high cholesterol); osteoarthritis (joint pain);
lower back pain; prescription renewal; gastro-esophageal reflux
disease (heartburn); gynecological examination; acute bronchi-
tis; asthma; and anxiety.

These top 14 reasons account for only a third of the reasons
people consult a family doctor. So imagine how much more
likely family doctors are to face questions they can't answer
than, say, doctors working in highly focused subspecialty practices like the glaucoma clinic Pierre visited.

Pierre has a favourite image he likes to use to illustrate the
difference between specialist and generalist physicians. Physicians with specialized practice are like commercial airline pilots.
They spend most of their days in very well-known territory, fly-
ing on autopilot. Family physicians with a general practice, on
the other hand, are more like bush drivers. They spend a lot of

their day navigating bumpy roads such as managing patients who have complex care needs (e.g., patients with multiple chronic diseases and mental health issues who are taking several medications and who lack the resources to cope with ill health and other stresses in their lives) in partnership with family caregivers and multidisciplinary teams. Maps are of little use to them because they aren't sure where they are a lot of the time.

Today, thanks to the Internet, family doctors have a kind of GPS that allows them to find their way through the bush. Many family physicians already see how radically the Internet can improve their work. As one doctor explained to Pierre, "I had a patient who suffered from obesity and wanted a medication to help with appetite suppression. You know, sometimes you just can't remember the name of a medication. Or you don't know where to look for it." But in this case, the doctor simply looked up obesity treatment on a site called Lexi-Drugs.

More and more, patients are starting to see the advantages of doctors searching for information during their consultations. Pierre recalls an interview with a family doctor who explained, "It's a funny thing … because often as a physician, if you're not sure of a medication and you look it up in your big blue paper book, the patient sometimes looks at you like, 'Oh, you know, she doesn't know what she's doing.' But when you look it up on your little hand-held computer, it is different and some patients may be like, 'Oh, she's into technology. She's up to date!'"

A lot of this huge potential is going to waste, and it's not just because the Internet makes some patients think doctors don't know what they are doing. There's something else family doctors are missing.

For many patients, it's not the technology that makes them feel uncomfortable. They simply want to feel assured that their clinician is consulting a reliable source. In other words, patients want to know what doctors are looking at.

By now, almost everyone who uses the Internet – and that's most people – knows that the quality (trustworthiness) of the information on the Internet can vary immensely: from the latest research to complete nonsense, or worse, information that is presented as being scientific research but is in fact just marketing. So, naturally, when patients watch their doctor, pharmacist, or nurse turn to the Internet for answers, many fear they might be surfing the web indiscriminately. Hence the "why is my doctor Googling it?" fear.

In the study we mentioned earlier that was published in *Canadian Family Physician*, researchers found that about a third of patients do not like it when their doctor looks for information during a consultation, unless the doctor tells them they are using a specialized medical resource.[5] This finding wasn't restricted to the Internet. Information sources could be medical textbooks or other resources, as long as they were specifically for use by doctors.

When their doctors explained they were consulting a reliable source, only 9% of patients said their confidence in their physician decreased and only 7% thought they were getting a lower quality of care. In other words, people don't mind clinicians looking things up in front of them, as long as they know they are searching for information from a reliable source.

Strangely, doctors don't seem to be aware of this concern, as half of the 54 family doctors who participated in this exploratory study said they believed patients preferred not to know where doctors were looking for information. A third of the doctors said they expected patients to report negative perceptions about the quality of their care if they knew where their doctor was looking for information.

Every year, thousands of articles are published in scientific and professional journals on common diseases like diabetes and in trendy areas like genomics. In comparison, little has been written, at least so far, about how electronic knowledge resources can improve the work of family physicians and other professionals in primary health care, such as nurses, nurse practitioners, and community pharmacists.

Most of what has been written about family doctors has focused on practice improvement. The reigning philosophy is that doctors should find and apply practice guidelines and use the best available evidence they have for their patients, taking into account the uncertainty of research results and the clinical situation of their patients.

It's a shame there is so little interest in how electronic knowledge resources can improve the work not only of doctors but also of nurses and pharmacists. Clinicians are human and can make mistakes on the basis of what they know or do not know. If they access these resources they can reduce the number of mistakes they make, thereby improving quality of care and patient safety.[6]

That's not all. Given the enormous expansion of information and the continuous development of information and communication technology, most medical knowledge is now located mainly in electronic knowledge resources. As a result, doctors need to be comfortable using the Internet to look things up. It's the only way they will stay up to date.

Things are changing. In recent decades, doctors have been taught to recognize that there are many uncertainties in caring for patients. They have learned to look at the grey zones and come up with concrete questions about specific cases for which they can then seek answers.

But doctors need to go further. With so much information available today, they need to start considering the process of diagnosing patients and managing health care plans as a learning process. They have to start looking at their daily work not as holding a whole bunch of information in their heads but as part of their lifelong learning.

In his work with residents and students, Roland likes to quote the British doctor Sir Muir Gray (director of the National Knowledge Service in the United Kingdom and chief knowledge officer of the National Health Service), who said, "The application of what we already know will have a bigger impact on health and disease than any drug or technology likely to be introduced in the next decade."[7]

How can patients and family caregivers help to get their doctors to change their thinking? This book is for everyone, and we suggest a simple first step: Tell your clinician that you think "looking it up" is a good thing, and ask them to recommend high-quality electronic knowledge resources (e.g., relevant online consumer health information) and to show you how to look it up by yourself or with someone else (e.g., a relative with health training or a health librarian) if necessary.

Chapter 2

Do I Really Need This Test?

Paul, a tall, handsome 55-year-old, was a successful, prominent businessman. He had been a regular patient of Roland's for years. An avid tennis and golf player, he looked robust and healthy. He always arrived for his visit with an optimistic, level-headed attitude about his health.

But this time, Roland could tell that something was amiss. Roland began by asking Paul the routine question: Had he had any health problems since his last visit? Paul said he hadn't, but something in his voice suggested otherwise. So Roland probed.

As Roland would soon learn, Paul had lost his father to lung cancer since his last visit. Since Paul was a smoker himself, his father's death had been a double shock. The risks of smoking had suddenly become very real. When Roland finished taking Paul's blood pressure, Paul asked if he should have a CT scan of his chest to screen for lung cancer, "just in case."

Lung cancer is the second most common type of cancer among both men and women, and it is the leading cause of cancer death in the United States; in 2015, there were more than 220,000 new cases of lung cancer (more than 13% of all cancer cases).[1]

Given this, one might assume that early detection is important. In 2002, the American College of Radiology decided to look at whether early detection actually was decreasing the number of deaths from lung cancer. That year, it launched a randomized controlled trial called the National Lung Screening Trial that followed almost 54,000 current or former heavy smokers in 33 medical centres in the United States. In 2011, the American College of Radiology released its findings: CT scans were associated with a 20% relative decrease in death from lung cancer.

In the wake of this trial, the US Preventive Services Task Force (USPSTF), an independent group of national experts that makes recommendations about clinical preventive services, recommended that anyone 55 to 80 years old who currently smokes or who smoked at least one pack of cigarettes per year for 30 years (and who has smoked within the past 15 years) should be screened for lung cancer.

Roland knew about this recommendation. He also knew a CT scan might be reassuring for Paul. Who knew what they would find? It might save his life.

There was just one hitch: Roland recalled that the number of false positives for lung cancer tests was particularly high. So he decided to see if Paul's situation really merited screening.

The information wasn't hard to find. When we think of doctors, we probably think of appointments before we think of apps. But that is about to change. Apps have enormous potential for allowing doctors to quickly get the information they need to diagnose and treat patients. Roland pulled out his mobile phone to do a quick check on an app the USPSTF provides on their website, called ePSS. After downloading the USPSTF app onto his smartphone, all Roland had to do was enter Paul's age and sex, click on "tobacco user" and "sexually active," and hit the start button to see what the recommendation was.

The USPSTF app categorizes its recommendations for providing a service such as a screening CT scan from "recommended" to "recommended against." In a few seconds, the app said Paul had a Grade B recommendation for CT scanning. That meant that if Paul was offered a CT scan there was a better possibility of benefit than of harm.

However, Roland wasn't quite ready to go ahead and recommend that Paul be screened. Roland knew that the USPSTF recommendation was at least a few years old so he decided to check to see if it was still valid. Like many members of the Canadian Medical Association, Roland receives (by daily email) regular updates of new clinical research called POEMS (this is an acronym for patient oriented evidence that matters).

Roland was glad he checked his POEMS. One of them had alerted doctors to a study that cast doubt on the USPSTF recommendation on CT screening for lung cancer. The POEM noted that one common concern about the USPSTF recommendations was that many positive results from the CT scans were actually false positives.

How can a positive result on a scan be false?

For some medical problems there is no such thing as a false positive. If you have an X-ray to find a bullet in your leg and the X-ray shows a bullet, there's no chance of a false positive (a bullet is seen, and there is a bullet). But for other conditions – notably cancers – the rate of false positives can be quite high (a cancer is suspected, but there is no cancer). False positives are actually a common problem in diagnostic testing. In the national lung cancer screening trial, about 95% of lung cancer screening results were false positives: "Across the three rounds, 96.4% of the positive results in the low-dose CT group and 94.5% of those in the radiography group were false positive results."[2]

The high rate of false positives means that when a test is used in the general population, it will cause harm for some people (we'll explain why in a moment). When these harms were taken into account, the net benefit of lung cancer screening turned out to be so small that the US Medicare program initially decided it would not pay for the tests. What's more, an American advisory panel concluded that even for individuals at high risk of lung cancer, the benefits of annual low-dose CT scans did not outweigh the harms.

Roland told this to Paul. Then he explained how a CT screen could be harmful. CT scans for screening expose patients to small doses of radiation, but they are not considered harmful because of that. The problem is that they result in a high number of false positives. After a positive CT scan, patients are sent to have a biopsy. A lung biopsy is a risky procedure, much more risky, say, than a biopsy for breast cancer. Lung biopsies involve sticking a needle directly into the lung. This can result in bleeding or infection that can land a patient back in the hospital. Even biopsies without complications are disruptive to people's lives. They cause worries that can last until all testing is complete, and that can sometimes take months, depending on the urgency of the condition, the type of surgery, and where the hospital is located.

Roland explained to Paul what he had found: there was a recommendation from the USPSTF to screen, but it was controversial and a test with a false positive could land him in the hospital. Paul appreciated being made aware of the risks. In the end, he decided not to have a CT scan. Instead of spending time getting screened, he decided to finally quit smoking.

All of this happened in one 20-minute appointment, thanks to Roland's smartphone and an app.

Other apps help doctors and patients make sense of test results and decide whether treatment is the best course of action in that patient's situation. High cholesterol is a good example as it is a common concern for middle-aged people at risk of heart disease. Most doctors have their patients get their cholesterol levels tested. Patients then want to know if their cholesterol level is good or bad.

However, contrary to what has become a common belief, there is actually no normal level of cholesterol. The risk of heart disease depends on the relationship between cholesterol and other factors for each individual patient. Doctors can figure that out in a few seconds by using an app, such as the one available at http://chd.bestsciencemedicine.com/calc2.html. The doctor enters a patient's age, sex, and blood pressure and indicates whether the patient smokes or has diabetes. The app then predicts the chance that the patient will develop heart disease in the next 10 years.

How accurate is the app? Its algorithms are based on conclusions from one of the most famous epidemiological studies ever carried out: the Framingham Heart Study. The study has followed 5,209 adult subjects from Massachusetts since 1948, and it is still going on. Much of the common knowledge we have today about heart disease – like the effects of diet, exercise, and even common medications like aspirin – were early discoveries of this study, whose later findings included the role of smoking, cholesterol, and blood pressure. In short, the app uses trustworthy information from scientific research and makes calculations using validated algorithms.

The goal of this story is not to discourage people from asking for tests. Our point is that preventive tests are not always beneficial, and they can sometimes be harmful. With the electronic knowledge resources that doctors have – literally – at their fingertips today, doctors can find exactly the information their patients need to help them decide whether to have a test (or not).

This ability to find information is more important than ever, because more patients are asking for preventive tests than ever. Why? People hear about tests from headlines, or relatives, or someone who has a concern or condition similar to their own. Or they hear about a celebrity who is recommending being checked for a specific disease; for instance, comedian Rosie O'Donnell and Nancy Reagan have endorsed mammograms, Rudy Giuliani has claimed that screening for prostate cancer saved his life, and TV host Katie Couric recommended getting a colonoscopy after losing her husband to colon cancer. Just hearing about a test makes people wonder whether they should have it.

There is also a deeper reason that more and more people are asking for preventive tests: people have come to think of such tests as part and parcel of their annual checkup. In fact, the very idea of an annual checkup is relatively recent, and these days it's under considerable scrutiny among health services experts and experts in the primary health care community. Their thinking is that we can take the time and energy we would have invested in screening people without symptoms and instead help those people who actually have symptoms.

The yearly examination has only been part of our medical routine since the 1970s. Before that, people saw doctors when they were sick or if they were rich enough to afford to visit them. Until 1957, hospital services in Canada were private. In Quebec, health care services were private until 1970, when Quebec's provincial health insurance program was put in place. Until Obamacare was introduced in the United States, being hospitalized or treated for chronic disease in that country was a major cause of debt, because only rich people or people with insurance (e.g., company coverage, individual insurance, Medicare for the elderly, Medicaid for the poor) had easy access to health care services.

The idea of an annual checkup did not come about because of common wisdom or for scientific reasons. Both Canada and the United States created government task forces to scrutinize the practice (the Canadian Task Force on Preventive Health Care and the USPSTF), and they discovered that the once-a-year custom has more to do with convenience than medical necessity. The one-year time interval was easy for patients to remember.

Having a checkup is not in itself a bad idea. The problem is that since the 1970s, medical organizations and some prominent medical doctors have oversold the importance of preventive medicine by spreading the idea that everyone needs to have preventive tests during an annual medical checkup. Most doctors and patients believe that early detection of disease is always better, so this reinforces the belief that it is wise and cost-effective to have annual checkups.

But this is not necessarily true. One reason is that medical diagnostic techniques have become so advanced and so sensitive that doctors can – and do – detect "diseases" that in some cases will never cause harm to patients.

One US doctor has become a particularly outspoken critic of the annual checkup. Gilbert Welch, a professor of medicine at the Dartmouth Institute for Health Policy and Clinical Research, wrote a book with Lisa Schwartz and Steve Woloshin called *Overdiagnosed: Making People Sick in the Pursuit of Health*. As Welch explained in an interview, "The place where I have a problem, and where I think a lot of doctors have a problem, is when you have this vision of an annual check-up where we really look hard to see if we can find something wrong."[3]

According to Welch, not only is there little science to back up the annual checkup, more importantly, there is no scientific justification for a healthy person with no symptoms to have tests. He notes that "we all have abnormalities and our diagnostic capabilities are increasingly able to find them." At the most, he says, people shouldn't go for a periodic checkup; they should just check in occasionally with a doctor. "It should not be a concerted effort to look for things that are wrong."

Don't get us wrong – doctors aren't trying to deceive people by pushing the annual checkup. People (policy-makers, clinicians, and patients) have simply come to believe they need to have certain tests on a regular basis. Unfortunately, in many cases, a kind of routine has set in where otherwise healthy people without symptoms feel they need to make an annual visit to the doctor for blood tests and X-rays that offer little or no benefit and carry a real risk of harm. In fact, the number of tests anyone needs depends on their age, sex, family history, and other factors that are specific to each individual.

Why do doctors go along with this? Health professionals are professionals, so they apply rules. Otherwise, they risk being scrutinized by their professional organization. There is also social pressure from peers, magazines, and society in general to do things a certain way. Doctors, like patients, are not necessarily conscious of when they do things because of social norms and when they do them because of science and medicalization of the society. They can act without thinking critically. Patients may ask for a checkup, and doctors will agree as long as this is seen as standard practice. If the standards change – and they are changing – doctors and patients will change their behaviour, but this takes time.

Curiously, Pierre recently found himself automatically excluded from the patient list of the clinic he normally goes to. The reason was that he had not consulted his doctor for more than five years. When Pierre called for an appointment, the secretary told him that she assumed he had found another family physician and had archived his chart. She told him she expected patients to come to the clinic at least once a year for something, or every three years for a checkup. She did not see five years without a visit as a sign of a healthy client but rather she concluded the patient either was dead or had changed doctors. This is a strong – and unfortunate – cultural trait of contemporary health services. Either you consult periodically or clinics assume you have left or died. Cultural change takes time, so the new generation of medical secretaries may see things differently in the future.

Doctors' salaries play into the current culture. Health economists have repeatedly demonstrated that doctors (like everyone else) have financial expectations and find ways to meet those expectations. Sometimes doctors achieve their financial goals by doing more than they should. Insurance companies and health agencies also have financial expectations and are known to increase the number of some services or decrease others to meet these.

Again, medical diagnostic techniques are so advanced and so precise that doctors can – and do – detect diseases that in some cases will never cause patients harm. Breast cancer is a good example. Current knowledge is that breast cancer can be overdiagnosed. Researchers Archie Bleyer from the Oregon Health

& Science University and Gilbert Welch from the Dartmouth Institute for Health Policy and Clinical Research decided to take a look at the last 30 years of screening for breast cancer. In an article they published in the *New England Journal of Medicine*, they concluded that "more than 1.3 million women have been over-diagnosed in the past 30 years, roughly one in four breast cancers." Those cancers, they claimed, were "unlikely to have ever harmed the woman in the first place."[4]

But there's more, the researchers said. These overdiagnosed cancers "are a significant source of harm," the authors wrote, "since these patients face the burden of treatment, its adverse effects, and the psychological harm of living with a cancer diagnosis."

Online medical resources (such as choosingwisely.org) offer doctors lots of trustworthy and quickly assessable information they can use to avoid overdiagnosing, sparing patients from having to waste time, resources, and energy getting tests they don't need.

Jane was a self-confident 45-year-old lawyer. Her sister had been diagnosed with celiac disease, better known as gluten intolerance. During a visit, she asked her family doctor, Angela, an experienced 60-year-old physician whom Jane had been consulting for years, whether she should get tested.

Angela wasn't sure how to answer. "The patient was asking about whether some minor symptoms from her gastrointestinal tract could have been caused by celiac disease. And she was asking me about doing the testing. She had this family member and she wanted to know whether she could have the same problem, you know, because there's a genetic association."

Angela wasn't sure it was useful to do a test on someone who had minimal symptoms. So she decided to look it up.

What is celiac disease? The website of the Mayo Clinic – a highly respected source of medical and consumer health information that anyone can consult – offers a short explanation. For reasons that have not yet been well established, some immune systems overreact to gluten in food. The immune reaction "damages the tiny, hair-like projections (villi) that line the small intestine. Villi absorb vitamins, minerals and other nutrients from the food you eat." When these are damaged, the body is unable to absorb nutrients necessary for health and growth.

One of the reasons Jane asked for a test for celiac disease was that she had the impression it was becoming a more common disease, so there was a better chance she had it. Jane was partly right. Celiac disease is not very rare. It affects roughly one in 100 people, causing symptoms ranging from diarrhea and weight loss to anemia, fatigue, skin and dental problems, headaches, joint pain, and acid reflux (heartburn).

Pierre was curious about this perception. He went back to the Mayo Clinic website, which stated that the precise cause of celiac disease isn't known. "Some gene variations appear to increase the risk of developing the disease. But having those gene variants doesn't mean you'll get celiac disease, which suggests that additional factors must be involved." The website also noted that "sometimes celiac disease is triggered – or becomes active for the first time – after surgery, pregnancy, childbirth, viral infection or severe emotional stress."

The reason celiac disease *appears* to be getting more common is that people are hearing about it more. In recent years an increasing number of gluten-free products have been launched, including gluten-free foods, cookbooks, and advice books. Some celebrities are participating in this growing industry, notably actress Gwyneth Paltrow.

To make a decision about whether to recommend that Jane be tested, Angela went online and did a search for celiac disease in the Evidence-based Medicine Guidelines, a resource providing thousands of summaries of research findings. All doctors have to do is enter a search term, and in minutes they will find the information they need in a small number of short, easy-to-read paragraphs.

In a few minutes, Angela learned it was still unclear whether people without symptoms of celiac disease should be tested. Some experts (e.g., health economists and public health specialists) do not recommend mass screening or the screening of asymptomatic people.[5] In their view, the data just don't support it. Other experts (e.g., gastroenterologists) recommend screening all high-risk patients, such as the first-degree relatives of people with celiac disease.[6] There is no consensus on the issue.

By looking online, Angela also learned that a blood test can be used for initial screening for high-risk people such as first-degree relatives of patients with celiac disease. The blood test would be quick and simple, but Angela would need to be careful when interpreting the results from the test in someone who had no symptoms. "Finding out whether you have celiac disease is not as simple as having a blood test," she explained to Jane. Why? The test for celiac disease is among those that have a high rate of false-positive – but also false-negative – results.

If Jane had a positive result, the next step would be for her to have an endoscopy and a biopsy of the small intestine. The procedure is not very risky, but it is painful. Some patients can't stand the pain and have to come back at a later date to have the procedure done under anesthesia.

The good news about celiac disease is that it is treatable. Patients need to follow a gluten-free diet that completely eliminates wheat. But a biopsy of the small intestine would be a major endeavour for Jane, considering that she didn't have any symptoms of celiac disease, just a possible genetic predisposition.

Angela had a hunch it might not make sense for Jane to be tested right away. "I just basically repeated the information to her as I understood it. Just because you have a positive test doesn't mean that you have the disease—that's the message that I gave her."

But the decision was up to Jane. After Angela quickly summarized what she had learned, Jane decided not to go ahead with further testing. Going through the complete diagnostic process was more complicated than she had imagined, with more uncertainties. She didn't think it was worth the time and stress involved, especially since experts didn't even agree it was worthwhile for someone without symptoms to be tested in the first place.

There is still no medical consensus about whether we should screen for celiac disease in high-risk people without symptoms. The recommendation in the 2008 guidelines not to screen patients without symptoms still holds, and screening people without symptoms is usually not recommended. In fact, this is an example of a classic medical controversy where specialists promote testing while public health experts say the evidence for such testing isn't there. Although specialists claim to be acting in the interests of public health, their recommendations put them in a conflict of interest, since testing boosts the prestige of their discipline.

For many people, the idea of watching a doctor do a Google search in front of them during a medical consultation sounds, well, crazy. But it won't seem crazy for long if useful searches (as in Angela's story) become just another way of solving problems that arise in everyday practice. More and more doctors are doing this.

However, when doctors turn to their computers or pull out their mobile devices, it's usually not to search Google or use any other generic search engine. Doctors who look for information in front of their patients generally know what they are looking for and on which site(s) they are likely to find it.

People will get used to watching doctors like Angela looking things up. But first, they need to understand how doctors having quick and easy access to trustworthy information can – and should – change the relationship they have with their doctor.

In the traditional, paternalistic model of medical care, the one most of us are used to, the doctor serves as an active expert and the patient is expected to be more or less passive.

Physicians make decisions and patients do "what the doctor ordered," as the old expression goes.

But this scenario is changing. Slowly but steadily, the traditional doctor-patient encounter is giving way to a new type of communication between doctors and patients. We could call this the Medical Consultation Version 2.0. Researchers and doctors call this new model shared decision-making. The movement toward this model was started, and is still led, by clinician-researchers (doctors who do part-time research).

What is shared decision-making? First of all, it is appropriate in cases where a patient has a choice between equally acceptable options – usually, having a test or a treatment, or not. When clinicians and patients find themselves in this situation – and they often do – patients engaged in shared decision-making do not expect a categorical answer when they ask a question. Instead, they ask their clinician a question, and the clinician becomes a source of information that both patient and clinician use to make a decision together about the next steps.

In shared decision-making, clinicians provide information, or they find it if they don't have it. Then they discuss with their patient the benefits and risks of sticking to the status quo and the benefits and risks of having a test or starting a new treatment. Simply put, clinicians can look for information on a condition, explain what they found to their patients (both positive and negative aspects), then share the decision-making with their patient by engaging the patient in a discussion about what they think.

We work with two world leaders in the field of shared decision-making, from Laval University: France Légaré and Holly Witteman. One important point they stress in their research and writing is that shared decision-making can only happen when there are equally acceptable options available.[7] If a doctor actually knows that one option is better than another, then shared decision-making isn't applicable. In such a case, the doctor should not hesitate to make a recommendation to the patient.

TABLE 1 TYPES OF PATIENT-CLINICIAN INTERACTIONS

| | TYPE OF PATIENT | | | |
Clinician interaction	Clinician role	Patient role	Information exchange	Goal
Paternalistic decision-making	Directive	Passive	One way (from clinician to patient)	Compliance of patient with clinician's rec-ommendation
Informed decision-making	Directive	Informed and informative	Two way (from clinician to patient, and vice versa)	Consensus between clinician and patient
Shared decision-making	Informative	Informative	Two way (from clinician to patient, and vice versa)	Equipoise (equity in the decision-making process)

Adapted from C. Charles, A. Gafni, and T. Whelan, "Decision-Making in the Physician-Patient Encounter: Revisiting the Shared Treatment Decision-Making Model," *Social Science and Medicine* 49, no. 5 (1999): 651–61, doi:10.1016/S0277-9536(99)00145-8.

Situations where there are equally acceptable options occur frequently in medicine and primary care, probably more often than most patients think. In such cases, Légaré writes, all of the health professionals involved and the patient (including their relatives and caregivers) should talk about the potential decision, "referring to the best available evidence and deliberating upon the consequences of each option," while respecting the patient's values and preferences.[8]

Table 1 illustrates three different scenarios adapted from a conceptual framework proposed by Cathy Charles (professor emeritus at McMaster University) and colleagues.[9] In the traditional paternalistic scenario, clinicians are seen as experts having sufficient information and power to impose a decision, which can be accepted (or not) by patients and their relatives. In the informed decision-making scenario, clinicians provide information to their patients and their relatives and then together they reach consensus about what seems to be the best option. In the shared decision-making scenario, clinicians and patients are seen as having complementary expertise and equal power because there is no best option. In this situation the principle of clinical equipoise applies: there is genuine uncertainty in the research and expert community over the benefits of a preventive intervention, diagnostic procedure, treatment, or referral. The clinician and patient exchange information and deliberate about the pros and cons of different possible options.

The shared decision-making movement started in Europe (with Glyn Elwyn, formerly from Wales and now teaching at Dartmouth College). Shared decision-making is now being widely adopted and promoted in Canada, Germany, the Netherlands, the United Kingdom, and the United States, among other countries. Numerous studies have shown that it improves patient health and can help to control health care costs. Specifically, shared decision-making can result in fewer hospital admissions, fewer elective surgeries, and lower costs for patients.[10]

Of course, to engage in shared decision-making, doctors need to have the necessary information at hand. That's where electronic knowledge resources come in. Interestingly, these resources have also been found to help patients feel more confident about engaging in shared decision-making with their doctors.

In a 2008 study, the Internet was already found to be working as a tool for advancing the practice of shared decision-making in medicine.[11] The researchers conducted focus groups with 16 volunteers, exploring their reasons for using online health information. The study asked them what they used the Internet for, whether they had looked for specific information on a health website, and whether they trusted the information they had found.

The findings suggested that using online information helps patients feel empowered. It gives them the background they need to better understand their clinicians' recommendations or to look into alternative treatments for themselves. As the authors of the study explained, despite their different educational and professional backgrounds, all of the participants in the study shared some opinions. They "enjoyed the immediacy of eHealth information," and the availability of eHealth information "empowered participants to make sense of their own experiences of health and illness which could act as a comfort whilst awaiting advice from a health professional."

On a summer day, Britney, a young family physician, saw Bernadette, a dynamic 60-year-old bank employee who liked doing physical exercise and was an avid volunteer. Bernadette was anxious about ovarian cancer. Her mother had had this type of cancer and she wanted to know if there was any blood test you could do to check for ovarian cancer.

Britney didn't think such a test existed. "I told her that I didn't think so, that I thought the blood work that we used was more for following someone who had been diagnosed with cancer. But I told her I would look into it." In the meantime, Britney gave Bernadette a slip for all the blood work she would normally do anyway.

Cancer in the family always causes anxiety. The possibility of developing cancer was especially stressful for Bernadette. She had watched her mother struggle with, and ultimately die from, the disease.

Fortunately, ovarian cancer is not common – it's actually 10 times less common than breast cancer. But it is more lethal: half the women diagnosed with ovarian cancer die from it. In 2013, there were 22,240 new cases in the United States (2.8% of all women diagnosed with cancer) and 14,030 deaths. It's known as the "silent killer" because often there are no symptoms until the disease has progressed to an advanced stage. Given how lethal the disease is, relatives of people who have had ovarian cancer have a compelling reason to request a screening test.

On her first search on the National Cancer Institute website, Britney read that "screening for ovarian cancer has not been proven to decrease the death rate from the disease." The National Cancer Institute recommended "prompt visits for any health change" instead. But Bernadette was clearly a high-risk patient, so Britney decided to look a bit further.

Britney searched two electronic knowledge resources: Essential Evidence Plus and UpToDate. Both had information on a test called cancer antigen 125 (CA 125) that measures the level of a protein produced by ovarian cancer cells and released into the bloodstream. The test is done to monitor the disease, but it can also be used to diagnose it. "Before that, I had no idea this test was ever used for anything but disease management," Britney explained, adding that unless she had consulted these websites, she would not have ordered this test for screening.

On a further search, Britney learned that the test was controversial. No major cancer or women's health organization recommended screening for women at average risk: not the American College of Physicians, the American Cancer Society, the National Cancer Institute, the American College of Obstetricians and Gynecologists, or the American Medical Women's Association. The test had a high rate of both false-positive and false-negative results.

Furthermore, on the website of the American Society of Clinical Oncology, Britney read the results of a study that followed patients at screening centres starting in 1993. The study found that CA 125 screening didn't reduce mortality – the proportion of women who were screened annually and died of ovarian cancer was the same as the proportion of women who hadn't been screened and died of this form of cancer.

However, Bernadette felt she was at above-average risk for ovarian cancer. Britney explained to her what she had found. "I gave her a lot of information. I spoke about the results you can get, and how it's not a perfect test. I explained that there's a high false-positive rate, and that if we got a positive [result] we would have to do other tests."

Britney herself felt the information she had found justified sending her patient for investigation. But she knew this was a situation where only shared decision-making would make sense. She also explained the uncertainty to Bernadette. "If it comes back positive, it doesn't mean you have cancer. It just means we have to look a little further." She explained the risks: namely, surgical removal of both ovaries in the case of early discovery.

Bernadette weighed the options and decided to go ahead with the test, so Britney ordered it. "It was reassuring for her to know that we will be keeping an eye on the possibility that she might be developing an ovarian cancer. By offering her the test now, I am going to screen her and hopefully prevent a disease."

Chapter 3

When Clinicians Disagree

"You should see this girl! She is absolutely stunning. She looks like a model and she's got all these kids and she's a great mother." Clara, a 50-year-old rural family physician in a small-town hospital, was particularly taken with the case of Rachel, a 32-year-old woman who was pregnant with her fifth child.

Rachel knew exactly what kind of birth she wanted. She had had two normal vaginal deliveries but had required a Caesarean section when she delivered twins after her last pregnancy. For this, her fourth delivery, she really wanted to have a vaginal birth. Part of the reason was that knowing how long it took to recover from a Caesarean section, she didn't have time for the procedure when she had four other small children at home.

Clara sympathized with Rachel. She was the mother of two teenagers herself and an active community member engaged in local organizations and politics. She was inspired by Rachel's energy and commitment and sympathetic to her desire to avoid another Caesarean section, especially if it wasn't necessary. But Clara knew a promise of a vaginal birth would be hard to "deliver" on.

"The facility I was working in did not, as a rule, do VBAC [vaginal birth after Caesarean]," Clara explained in our interview. "Patients who wanted one were usually transferred to a referral centre about an hour and 10 minutes away." Indeed, Clara "got a lot of flak from the nurses at the hospital" when she proposed a VBAC for Rachel, she said. "They were afraid that I was putting them in an unsafe situation."

Clara herself was quite sure that Rachel could have a safe vaginal birth. She knew that the traditional position on VBAC – that it was not a safe option after a Caesarean section – had changed over time, thanks to research that had demonstrated it was safe under certain conditions. "I knew that the success rate of a planned vaginal birth in a woman with Rachel's clinical parameters was high," she said.

However, attitudes in the medical community haven't necessarily kept pace with new research. So, facing resistance from her hospital, Clara had two options: she could either transfer Rachel to another centre, which was neither her first choice nor Rachel's, or she could try to convince her colleagues to let Rachel deliver at the local hospital.

Clara decided to give the second option a shot. She explained to her colleagues that for someone like Rachel, who had a previous history of rapid, normal deliveries, putting her on the road for an hour and 10 minutes when she was in labour was not advisable. "There was a risk that she would have her baby in the car or in an ambulance."

But the nurses were still doubtful a vaginal birth at their hospital was the best option. So Clara decided to look it up to back her argument up with some research. "I wanted to have really good data so I could discuss the issue with the nurses and other physicians in my group," she explained. "I also wanted to get good data to discuss successes and failures and risks with Rachel."

At home, the night before her next appointment with Rachel, Clara did a search for a risk/benefit analysis of VBAC. She found two systematic literature reviews – syntheses of high-quality research evidence on specific medical questions – in the database Essential Evidence Plus. Each concluded that both planned elective repeat Caesarean section and planned induction of labour for women with a prior Caesarean birth had known benefits and harms. Both reviews noted that the conclusions needed to be interpreted with caution. In other words, there was no medical consensus about the risks versus benefits of a vaginal birth following a Caesarean birth.

Clara looked further. That's when she found a decision support calculator on the site of Essential Evidence Plus that could estimate the probability a woman would have a successful VBAC. The decision rule outlined different conclusions for three separate situations a woman might be in at the time of admission, depending on the degree of cervical effacement, which is a measurement taken as soon as women arrive at the hospital that estimates their progress in labour. Using the decision support calculator, Clara saw that Rachel would have a 95%, 93%, or 89% chance of having a successful vaginal birth, depending on her degree of cervical effacement when she arrived at the hospital. These high likelihoods were due mainly to the fact that Rachel had already had a vaginal birth and that she was young. "This just basically gave me some concrete numbers I could use."

After Clara explained to her colleagues what she had found online, they agreed to the VBAC for Rachel. The extra information was reassuring to the mother as well. "I explained to her some of the risks associated with it and why some of the other health care professionals had not been as cooperative," says Clara.

Months later, Rachel successfully delivered her fifth baby. "She had a completely normal vaginal delivery," said Clara. "She went home a happy lady the next day and three days later she went to a party! If she had had a Caesarean section, she would have had a much longer recovery."

But the story didn't end there. After Rachel's delivery, Clara decided to talk to her colleagues about the information she had found while treating Rachel. "I made my case that because of the nature of obstetrics, sometimes we have to be willing to provide a service when the alternative is not as safe," and "health care professionals can't always follow very strict rules; we have to be flexible with regard to the patient and the situation," she said.

The message got through. The information Clara found was later used to improve the hospital's obstetrical program.

Contrary to what you see on TV dramas, medical professionals who work together don't spend a lot of their time arguing with each other about cases. What they do frequently engage in are (less dramatic) "corridor consultations." These occur when doctors literally meet in the corridor, out of earshot of their patients, and discuss a specific patient problem.

Most doctors consider it an advantage – even a privilege – to be able to slip out of a consultation with a patient and discreetly get a second opinion from a colleague, especially when they are not sure of the best course of action. These sorts of consultations happen much more regularly than disagreements, and especially more frequently than open conflicts.

When disagreements between doctors do happen, if the doctors can turn to quickly accessible, reliable electronic knowledge resources they can resolve their disagreements much more easily.

There are a number of reasons a doctor might feel compelled to challenge a colleague's management of a patient. Medicine is often not based on science. Clinical practice guidelines, which doctors can use to inform their decisions, are not always based on a consensus of opinion reached after the writers of the guidelines have examined the evidence from multiple research studies. There is a lot of uncertainty. That's one reason medical decisions are not made automatically. Many factors enter into a doctor's decision, including the values of the patient and the personal experience of the doctor.

Doctors and patients can also disagree. Sometimes patients want tests they have heard about from a friend or relative, even if they have no symptoms and there's no medical reason for having the test. In rare cases, a patient may insist on having a test even when his or her doctor completely disagrees. Sometimes when patients aren't satisfied with the explanations from their doctor, they seek a second opinion or even a third opinion.

These disagreements, either between doctors or between doctors and patients, are not necessarily a bad thing, especially when clinicians take advantage of differences of opinion to "look it up." In doing this, doctors can essentially get a quick third opinion. If a doctor has doubts about a colleague's diagnosis or treatment of a particular case, he or she can find research to support his or her case in a matter of minutes, or even seconds. This allows colleagues to discuss the facts instead of (in the worst cases) fruitlessly sparring over interpretations or speculation.

Generally speaking, looking up a third opinion online leads to better treatment for patients. Disagreements are often resolved, for instance, when physicians directly consult research studies. Such studies don't dictate how a patient situation should be addressed. Rather, they inform doctors about the research that has been done on a condition or disease or a treatment. That information can then give more weight to one treatment option, or diagnosis, over another.

As we mentioned in the Introduction, a group of doctors initiated the evidence-based medicine movement some 25 years ago at McMaster University to encourage doctors to use research evidence (the results of current scientific research studies) when treating patients. It was hard to do back then, mostly because doctors had to go to libraries to find the latest research on diseases or treatments.[1] Over two decades later, readily available trustworthy medical information allows doctors, nurses, and pharmacists to find answers quickly, making it easier than ever to practise evidence-based medicine.

Like the Internet, research evidence has few borders. That means physicians across the planet can consult the same information. The Cochrane Reviews are a good example. Produced by the Cochrane organization (cochrane.org), they are available through the online Cochrane Library (cochranelibrary.com). Cochrane describes itself as a global network of 37,000 health practitioners, researchers, patient advocates, and other clinicians from 130 countries who produce trustworthy, accessible health information free from commercial sponsorship and other conflicts of interest.

The organization was named after Archie Cochrane (1909–1988), a British epidemiologist who advocated the use of scientific experiments (typically randomized controlled trials) as a basis for decision-making in medicine. The Cochrane Library claims to have no head office; instead, it operates out of 14 centres around the world including ones in Canada and the United States. Most of the work involved in creating and disseminating the reviews is carried out online.

The Cochrane Library provides systematic literature reviews that are considered the best evidence because they pool and synthesize the results of all of the scientific studies that have been conducted on the topic in question. Individual studies may produce conflicting recommendations (e.g., the results of one study may lead to a "treat" recommendation for a particular condition whereas the results of another may lead to a "don't treat" recommendation). If the results of all available studies are combined, however, the large pool of data will often reveal a statistically significant result that clearly supports either the "treat" or "don't treat" recommendation.

Sometimes, systematic literature reviews conclude that not enough high-quality studies have been conducted to warrant making a recommendation or that there is too much contradictory evidence among high-quality studies to support any particular recommendation. Systematic literature reviews don't necessarily offer simple answers to clinical questions, but they often provide evidence that doctors can use to decide in favour of one option over another and to estimate the benefits and harms of different options.

Of course, sometimes even this information leads to disagreements between doctors. Pierre worked on a study where researchers set out to see what kind of tensions arose from information found online – in this case, between family medicine residents and their supervising doctors.

Residents are doctors who have graduated from medical school but are still honing their craft during an intensive apprenticeship in clinical settings. For example, family medicine residents practise for at least two years under the supervision of senior family physicians. In Canada, residents must demonstrate to their superiors that they are competent in seven roles: as collaborator, communicator, family medicine expert, health advocate, manager, professional, and scholar.[2]

Most studies on the issue have shown that patients support the role of residents. For example, 265 patients completed a questionnaire while waiting in the office of four family physicians affiliated with a medical training program.[3] These patients indicated that there were two reasons they preferred being seen by family medicine residents: they liked "that they could contribute to training new doctors" and that they would "receive two opinions instead of one."

This doesn't change the fact that differences of opinion often arise between doctors and residents. In one such case, Charles, a resident working at a health clinic in a large French-speaking city, was seeing Christophe, an athletic 29-year-old man with a persistent ache in his knee. Christophe had already seen two doctors to try to figure out what the problem was and how to solve it. The doctors had each given him a categorical, but entirely different, answer. One had said he had tendinitis. The other had said it was knee pain with an unknown cause.

Christophe came to Charles to get a third opinion. "One doctor told me one thing and the other told me another. It just didn't make sense," Christophe explained. "And I still have pain."

When Christophe told the story of the consultations in detail, one element jumped out at Charles: Christophe mentioned that he had had Osgood-Schlatter disease when he was younger. Osgood-Schlatter is an irritation of the patellar ligament (the front face of the knee) at the tibial tuberosity (the small spike emerging from the front face of the bone situated about one inch under the knee). It commonly occurs in athletic teenagers and is thought to be caused by a combination of growing bones and excessive sports training. "Naturally I wondered if there was a connection between that condition and what he was experiencing now," Charles said.

Charles decided to look it up. "I could barely recall what I had learned about Osgood-Schlatter in medical school, so I told the patient I would go read up on it for a few seconds." Charles headed to the residents' room and looked up Osgood-Schlatter in two general electronic knowledge resources: UpToDate and the 5 Minute Clinical Consult, known as 5MCC, one of the seven resources included in the database of InfoRetriever (the original name of Essential Evidence Plus). "5MCC told me that the pain from Osgood-Schlatter can return in almost 50% of adults who suffered it as teenagers. No other site said that, and it got me thinking, is it an error?"

Things seemed to be getting more complicated, not less. Christophe had two unsatisfactory diagnoses from other doctors and now he had contradictory information from two different databases.

Charles decided to take the contradictory evidence to one of the orthopaedic specialists Christophe had consulted and see what she thought. "Osgood-Schlatter doesn't come back, exactly," she said. "Adults can have the same pain, but we don't call it Osgood-Schlatter. We just call it tendinitis." Charles realized that the 5MCC site was cutting corners a bit by saying the condition could come back in adults. "It can come back, but it comes back with a different name."

Charles explained to Christophe what he had found out – contradictions and all. "I told him I took a good look at the whole question. I like to be as honest as possible with patients and really do as much research as I can to be as thorough as possible. There are patients who really want a doctor to tell them, 'That's the disease. Here's the treatment.' But my clientele is pretty young and educated and they get the fact that medicine isn't 100%."

The treatment was the same in either case: anti-inflammatory medication. "But I mostly recommended reducing his activity and avoiding the specific activities that increased his pain."

The conflict around the best treatment for Christophe didn't change much, but it did make him feel better. "Christophe told me he was happy I hadn't pretended to know everything. At least he knew I wasn't just feeding him a line. He's had an honest answer to his questions. Someone really looked into it for him. If I hadn't been able to look it up, I would have treated him differently. I mean, I wouldn't have had a clue what Osgood-Schlatter even was [what it means for adults]!"

Pierre likes to say he practised in the last century. He actually began practising just a couple of decades ago, in the 1990s. But from Pierre's vantage point today, those really were the old days. Back then, Pierre kept reference books, professional journals, and a red pocketbook, which was a comprehensive manual of treatment recommendations (called the Dorosz), where he wrote notes updating information on drugs. He also tucked notes from medical school, from meetings with colleagues, and from articles he read in professional journals into the notebook.

Pierre referred to his red book at least once a day, to calculate drug doses for children according to their weight, for instance. The book was full of handwritten notes, and he had access only to information by drug type – for example, antibiotics. He did not have real-time access to treatment recommendations or general medical information on any topic, like he does today. Pierre only had to buy a new book every two years because drugs did not change that quickly – or so he thought.

Many top electronic knowledge resources are now updated, on average, once a year. But some Internet sites update their content immediately when new information, research results, or guidelines become available. Most resources that provide treatment recommendations have editors – either doctors or pharmacists – who are experts on a topic and responsible for each "chapter." This editor tracks and stays abreast of new information on the topic. A number of professionals in the field – usually volunteers – also find and submit new information. The entire resource is under the control of a team of health professional editors who maintain the consistency and coherence of the information and verify that it's valid. For example, RxTx (formerly e-Therapeutics+) is produced by a non-commercial professional organization (the Canadian Pharmacists Association) and combines resources on pharmacologic and non-pharmacologic treatment recommendations, minor ailments, drug-drug interactions, and information for patients and family caregivers. This is the equivalent of about five updated volumes of roughly 500 pages each, searchable from anywhere in the world with an Internet connection. It's the clinical tool Pierre dreamed of having in the 1990s: one that gives him current medical knowledge at his fingertips that he can pull up whenever he needs it.

It's fortunate that up-to-date information is so readily available today because clinicians will be more likely to disagree with each other as time goes on. The reason is simple: primary care clinicians work together more than ever in the past, and this trend will continue. Solo practice, a model in which individual doctors operate their own offices, is quickly becoming a model only some older doctors continue to use.

Over the last two decades, doctors throughout North America have been steadily moving toward group practices in which they work in multidisciplinary collaborative teams made up of doctors, nurses, dieticians, social workers, pharmacists, and other health professionals. These are typically called medical home or family health teams or groups. The idea is for professionals to provide comprehensive, accessible, and coordinated primary health care to meet the needs of the community they serve. This trend has been called primary care reform and is gaining momentum throughout North America.

In a study published in 2014 in the *International Journal of Family Medicine*, researchers found that in 1986–87, 51.8% of physicians in Canada worked in solo practices. In 1997, this figure had decreased to 31.3%, and by 2010, just 22.3% of physicians worked in this type of practice.[4] This trend is also happening in other countries, like the Netherlands, where the percentage of solo practitioners decreased from 67.4% in 1990 to 39.1% in 2010.[4]

Why are doctors teaming up? On the whole, they believe that group practices provide better quality care to patients, and many studies back this up. But there are advantages in it for health professionals too. When they have to be absent, they know someone else in their clinic can fill in for them, a scenario that is convenient for doctors and reassuring to patients.

Group practices are also the product of a big generational change in the medical community: today's doctors just aren't as willing to work long hours as their predecessors were. There are also more female doctors, and many of them (and young male doctors) take at least some time off to have and care for children.

But there is also another trend underway – though it might be more accurate to call it a philosophy – that encourages doctors to work together or at least to communicate better. Among health professionals, this is known as promoting continuity of care and refers to the goals of coordinating care by clinicians and health organizations. Continuity of care has two guiding principles: providing care over time and focusing on individual patients. In plain language, one could also call this making sure patients don't get bounced around in the system.

In mental health care, the clinician-patient relationship is typically established with a team rather than a single provider. In this field, continuity of care refers to ensuring the stability of patient-provider relationships over time. In nursing, continuity of care emphasizes information transfer and coordination of care over time, and communication between nurses. The goal is to maintain a consistent approach to care between nurses and to personalize care to the patient's changing needs during an illness."[5] Continuity of care, on the whole, is believed to reduce health care usage (e.g., the need for unnecessary emergency visits to the hospital) and increase quality of life and patient satisfaction.

No matter what the context, continuity of care requires good communication between medical professionals. Being able to quickly find trustworthy information can only help this. Experts call this informational continuity: good communication of patient-centred information among all clinicians involved in caring for a patient.

What it means in practice is that more clinicians will be "looking it up," getting more details about subjects about which they do not have in-depth knowledge and communicating this information to other clinicians who are involved in the care of a patient. It will mean, for example, that nurse practitioners working in medical teams will check specialized medical information reported in their patients' charts or use online information to address their doubts if they disagree with something. In short, even when "looking it up" leads to disagreements, thanks to the availability and accessibility of online medical information, these disagreements are bound to produce a win-win situation for patients.

One May morning, Charlotte, a new nurse practitioner, saw an 81-year-old man named Roger. One of her colleagues had seen the patient and diagnosed him with a transient ischemic attack, which produces stroke symptoms that disappear in less than a day. Before this incident, a doctor had put Roger on aspirin to prevent strokes. After the stroke, the doctor did not change his treatment.

Charlotte had doubts about this course of action. To prevent a future stroke, she wondered if she should tell Roger to continue taking aspirin, or stop the aspirin and start clopidrogel, another drug commonly used to prevent strokes. She knew there was also a third option: continue aspirin and also start clopidrogel.

Nurse practitioners, also known as advanced practice registered nurses (APRN), are not yet widely known in Canada. Their profession was created in the United States in the mid-1960s, in response to a shortage of medical doctors, especially in rural areas. There are presently about 4,000 nurse practitioners working in Canada (13 for every 100,000 people) and 56,000 in the United States (18 for every 100,000 people).[6]

Nurse practitioners do many of the things doctors do: they diagnose and treat illnesses, evaluate patients, and manage acute and chronic illnesses; they perform physical examinations and request X-rays, electrocardiograms (EKGs), or physiotherapy; and they assist in, or even perform, minor procedures like suturing. Research has repeatedly demonstrated that when nurse practitioners are present, they significantly reduce medical costs and improve health care services and patient health.[7]

Charlotte was still quite inexperienced when she faced this choice. "I'd never had to start such treatment on my own or prescribed a medication yet, so it was new for me."

The first thing she did was look it up. Charlotte searched e-Therapeutics+. "I went to see 'Prevention of ischemic stroke,' then 'Therapeutics Tips,' then 'Pharmacologic Choices.' After that I clicked 'clopidogrel' on 'Pharmacologic Choices.' That's where I saw the recommended dose. After that I could check the risks and benefits of leaving him on aspirin and clopidogrel at the same time."

Charlotte first found that "the combination of low dose aspirin and clopidogrel did not significantly reduce the rate of ischemic events including stroke in patients with recent stroke or transient ischemic attack (warning stroke) when compared with clopidogrel alone, or in patients with multiple risk factors when compared with low dose aspirin alone." In other words, either medication was as good on its own as it was combined with the other.

But upon looking further, she discovered that the first option (aspirin only) is appropriate for prevention of a *first* occurrence of a stroke, not *after* a transient ischemic attack. E-Therapeutics+ recommended clopidogrel only in the latter context.

Furthermore, combining the two drugs, Charlotte learned, "significantly increases the risk of bleeding in both trials and the risk of intracranial haemorrhage in the trial that enrolled patients with a history of stroke or TIA [transient ischemic attack]." The conclusion was that "the combination should not be used for long-term secondary prevention of ischemic events in patient with a history of stroke."

After checking with another physician and another online resource, Charlotte felt comfortable recommending that Roger take clopidrogel and stop aspirin. She then explained the information she found online to Roger and his wife. "I told them, 'It is you who must decide.'" Charlotte did not need to do much persuading. "Roger was pretty scared after his transient ischemic attack." But he was happy to hear exactly why the change in medication was being made.

In the long run, looking it up gave Charlotte the confidence she needed to make a decision on her own, even if it contradicted what a doctor had recommended. "You know, you're always second-guessing yourself," she says with a laugh. "I'd never had to initiate that therapy, so it was really something new for me. But now I can educate future patients about why we made that change in medication."

In some cases, patients themselves contribute to disagreements between clinicians. But again, when doctors use the disagreement as an opportunity to search for more information about a condition, everyone can benefit.

In August 2008, Claire, an experienced nurse practitioner and professional leader, saw Cara, a 19-year-old woman who was living with epilepsy. Cara had decided to consult a nurse practitioner because she needed contraception, but her case was more complicated than usual. The drug Cara was taking to prevent seizures, carbamazepine, had the side effect of reducing the effectiveness of estrogen – one of the main ingredients in birth control pills – and at the same time put her at risk of fetal abnormalities if she were to conceive. (As a side note, services such as Motherisk can be freely consulted by members of the public seeking to better understand and quantify the risks associated with medicines, such as carbamazepine, during pregnancy.)

Cara told Claire that effective contraception was essential for her but she was worried about the side effects of a stronger birth control pill: she knew that higher doses of estrogen commonly cause migraine headache and nausea. Claire was quite sure that Cara would have to take contraception with a higher than average dose of estrogen, so she referred her to a specialized epilepsy clinic. A doctor at the clinic recommended the same thing: Cara should take a contraceptive pill with a higher dosage of estrogen.

But Cara wasn't satisfied and decided to get yet another opinion, this time from a gynecologist. The gynecologist prescribed a contraceptive pill with a lower estrogen dose.

Claire knew this was risky. "The drug the gynecologist prescribed did not have the dose that is recommended. The gynecologist and I disagreed." So Claire decided to see if there was another option. She started by looking in e-Therapeutics+ to get more general information on epilepsy, as she had few patients with this condition. What did she find? "This information confirmed what I knew about birth control and the amount of extra estrogen needed. It had to be 35 micrograms. I was reassured that I wasn't giving this person too much and that this was absolutely the correct dose."

Claire explained her findings to Cara. "I knew it already, but I didn't have the details until I did my search. I encouraged Cara to stay on with the higher dose of estrogen. She didn't want to, but in the end, she accepted it."

Then Claire passed the information on to the gynecologist. "The whole thing was kind of good for me as I actually read through all the other details on epilepsy. The information confirmed what I did around birth control, and the amount of estrogen needed; I was reassured this was the correct thing to do."

Claire had just discovered one other great advantage of being able to quickly access medical research online. For clinicians, finding information depersonalizes a disagreement, making it easier to disagree in the first place.

As doctors in primary health care work more and more with other types of clinicians (nurses, pharmacists, psychologists, physiotherapists) in multidisciplinary teams, and personalities inevitably clash, having concrete information on hand can help avoid situations where one clinician refuses to listen to another. Valuable research-based information found online can quickly override professional disputes and rivalries. It's like a neutral third party.

After all, while constructive disputes are healthy, it's in everyone's interest to avoid unnecessary standoffs between clinicians.

Chapter 4

The Expanded Role of Pharmacists

Dave is a 35-year-old pharmacist in a community clinic. One afternoon he got a call from a physician he knew well at a nearby family health clinic. The physician's patient, a teenaged girl named Deborah, had been diagnosed with attention deficit and hyperactivity disorder (ADHD) on an earlier visit. Since that diagnosis, she and her parents had done some research about treatment.

Physicians at the clinic often called Dave about cases of older patients with several chronic diseases because their multiple medications increased the risk of drug interactions. This case was a bit different. The patient's parents had questions about a medication that their doctor couldn't answer. Even Dave wasn't sure. "I really needed to learn more about all of ADHD before I could even move forward," he explained.

No one knows exactly what causes ADHD. According to Statistics Canada, ADHD affects about 5% of the school-aged population in Canada and boys are three times more likely to develop it than are girls.[1] Individuals with the condition tend to act impulsively and have difficulty in social interactions. It's usually treated with a stimulant called methylphenidate, which helps reduce symptoms by increasing the concentrations of two hormones in the brain: dopamine and norepinephrine.

Deborah's parents did some research on ADHD after their daughter was diagnosed and read up on methylphenidate. They concluded that they didn't want their daughter to take this traditional stimulant; they wanted to try an alternative treatment instead. They arrived at their family physician's office with an article about atomoxetine, an alternative, non-stimulant medication used to treat ADHD.

Back 20 or even 10 years ago, when pharmacists had to go to libraries to get specialized information about new treatments just like physicians did, Dave might have been a bit taken aback by Deborah's parents. Looking up detailed information about a new alternative treatment used to be a time-consuming and not always fruitful endeavour.

But in this age of access to online information, Dave knew exactly what to do. "I remembered something about atomoxetine," he recalled. "There was some controversy about it and I knew it was relatively new to the market. Before I had a consultation with Deborah and her parents, I started looking into it."

Dave's first step was to log into the Pharmacist's Letter. When it was created in 1985, the Pharmacist's Letter really was a letter. Today, most pharmacists in the United States and Canada use it in its modern, online form. Like Cochrane synopses, the Pharmacist's Letter has short entries about medications with concise information that pharmacists (and some doctors) can quickly understand and apply.

The Pharmacist's Letter is a very popular resource among pharmacists, partly because it's clear and thorough. A quote by Albert Einstein hangs framed in the editorial staff's conference room: "If you can't explain it simply, you don't understand it well enough." The Pharmacist's Letter has a team of nine researchers who read the latest research studies on drugs then discuss the research with experts to make sure they understand it and, just as importantly, to make sure they can explain it correctly. (When pharmacists feel they need more information, they can consult the Detail-Documents section on the Pharmacist's Letter website, which has in-depth articles on specific questions and topics.)

The Pharmacist's Letter does more than explain new research: it's a truly interactive resource. Pharmacists who use the site submit thousands of questions each month. The staff narrows these down to about 350 topics per month then boils those down to roughly 35 "Big Questions" that their users are likely to face in daily practice. The information on the site ultimately goes through 14 editorial stages before it is published. In other words, staff at the Pharmacist's Letter figure out what information pharmacists *need* and then they use research studies to provide pharmacists with recommendations.

"The Pharmacist's Letter did a good job of detailing the drug itself," Dave explained, "and then I went to e-Therapeutics+ to read up on the management." This is what Dave found: "The efficacy of atomoxetine [an antidepressant] may be appropriate for those who have either not responded to, or not tolerated an adequate trial of stimulant medication." In other words, the alternative treatment was recommended as just that, an alternative.

When Dave met Deborah's parents, he knew he could give them valuable information and back up his recommendations with solid information. "Methylphenidate, not atomoxetine, is still the first-line treatment in ADHD. Atomoxetine is a relatively new drug and that means it shouldn't be used as a first-line treatment, especially for children. We don't know everything there is to know about that drug yet. I had to explain to the parents that yes, there is a place for atomoxetine in treating ADHD but that I felt we should start with what we know works for sure, which is methylphenidate. Then if it didn't work, we could move to atomoxetine." Dave printed the relevant patient leaflets from the Pharmacist's Letter and gave them to Deborah's parents to read.

Deborah's parents had done their research and appreciated the fact that Dave had been willing do to his too. They ended up accepting his recommendation. "Deborah is still coming back to her family doctor to adapt her dose and monitor effects. She's also seeing a counsellor, which is the first treatment for ADHD, and her case is evolving well," said Dave.

Like family physicians, pharmacists are seeing their practices change quickly with the arrival of more and more trustworthy online information.

"In my day, papers still existed," explains Silvia Duong, a dynamic young pharmacist who completed her doctoral training in 2007 and has been working as a clinical pharmacist in a large university hospital in a major Canadian city since 2011. We met her specifically to discuss whether more readily accessible medical information is changing the work of pharmacists today, and if so, how. Technologically speaking, Silvia knows that even though "her day" was only 10 years ago, in some ways it constitutes the old days. "The new generation of pharmacy students all have computers. They have to. Computers are fundamental to pharmacists' work," she says.

In fact, there's no way for pharmacists *not* to use computers. We're used to "looking it up," says Silvia. Pharmacists are a step ahead of doctors because they have been using electronic information for much longer. In community pharmacies, where pharmacists work behind the counter, drug information is built into the prescription processing system.

Online information is becoming more important than ever in pharmacists' work, for a number of reasons. First, there are more drugs available today than ever. Second, information about drugs and dosages is updated more frequently. When updates were published on paper, they were released about once a year. "Today, I want resources that have updates every four months, minimum," says Silvia.

The third reason pharmacists need to "look it up" more than ever is that the nature of their work is changing. When we were in medical school, in the 1980s, the role of pharmacists in physicians' work was barely mentioned: we learned to write prescriptions and expected pharmacists to fill them or call us if there was something wrong – end of story.

Things starting changing in the 1990s, after researchers began studying the impact pharmacists could have on helping manage patients, particularly those with multiple chronic conditions who required multiple medications. "Doctors often send me patients who are not responding to therapy or who are having drug interactions," confirms Silvia.

Today, more and more pharmacists work in family health clinics alongside doctors and nurses. Silvia is a member of an interdisciplinary family health team that includes family doctors, social workers, psychologists, and a nursing team. "Older patients, especially, are more likely to see different physicians. Each physician just adds on to the medications. From a crude point of view, before you know it, patients are on 20 medications. And that's when they send the case to me!"

In the medical world, this multiplication of medications is known as polypharmacy. Polypharmacy is usually defined as a situation in which a patient is taking five or more drugs. That's not at all uncommon today, as the population ages. In Canada, for instance, nearly two out of three seniors (62%) take five or more drugs, and almost one out of three seniors 85 years or older (29%) take at least 10 drugs.[2]

As the number of medications increases, so does the possibility the drugs will interact. A review of 11 research studies showed that about one in four seniors (over age 65) were taking at least one inappropriate drug.[3] This issue does not concern only seniors. In 2015, the Quebec Health and Welfare Commissioner warned professionals and the public that polypharmacy is increasing dramatically among non-elderly adults in North American and European countries.[4] For example, in Quebec more than half of adults (55%) regularly take medications (40% regularly take two or more drugs). That's why it's becoming more important, and more common, for pharmacists to act as doctors' partners rather than simply fill prescriptions that doctors write.

The pharmacists' role is also shifting because family health teams are becoming more common in family medicine. The trend is called inter-professional collaboration, and it's a long way from what doctors learned about the doctor-pharmacist relationship back in the 1980s.

How does this new collaboration work? Ontario provides a good example. Ontario's Family Health Team Initiative is a government program that has established some 200 teams across the province. Designed around specific community needs, these teams consist of family physicians, nurse practitioners, nurses, and sometimes chiropractors, rehabilitation workers, social workers, dieticians, pharmacists, other specialized physicians such as psychiatrists, and mental health workers.[5] These teams are similar to medical homes where a team of health care professionals provides health care from womb to tomb, as the expression goes. Research has shown that medical homes, compared with other types of primary care services, provide better access to health care, increase patient satisfaction with care, and improve health on the whole.

From a doctor's perspective, there are pros and cons to the new autonomy that pharmacists have. Proactive pharmacists can create new tensions or even conflicts with doctors, like the ones we discussed in the previous chapter. But as we have already seen, differences of opinion, when combined with reliable access to information, often bring about positive results in patient treatment and care.

Roland, for one, has seen pharmacists steadily become more autonomous and has seen both sides of the coin. On the down side, pharmacists sometimes hand patients sheets with every possible side effect of a medication. In doing so, they sometimes provoke false alarms by planting doubt in patients' minds. That can undermine the doctor's relationship with their patient.

However, Roland believes, like many physicians, that the benefits when pharmacists are proactive usually outweigh the harms. Pharmacists often catch mistakes, like wrong dosages and the potential for drug-drug interactions. They can suggest alternative drug treatments that interact less with other medications.

Contrary to what we, as physicians, were taught about the role of pharmacists when we were in medical school in the 1980s, today's pharmacists are sometimes involved in training residents. A national survey of family medicine residency programs revealed that one out of four (25.3%) training sites have pharmacist teachers.[6] When these teachers were questioned, more than 90% reported regularly searching for information on behalf of residents and teaching them about pharmacology and drug prescribing.

Of course, pharmacists aren't the only ones becoming more autonomous. Patients are less and less inclined to just follow the doctor's orders. They question doctors' authority more often than they used to. They want to hear the specific evidence for a doctor's decision. Of course, almost all also look up information on their own.

Pharmacists face the same challenges. Silvia Duong calls it the Dr Google effect. "Patients can look up information on their own, and they do! They get their own ideas about medication. Often they even decide they don't want to take medications."

There are, of course, advantages to having Dr Google there, Silvia admits. "I work in a clinic with lots of immigrants, people from all over the world. Sometimes they have been taking a medication in another country. Because of the language barrier, or sometimes just because I have never heard of it, I have trouble figuring out what it is. So I use Google myself! Sometimes I don't know how to spell the medication, but with Google, it's not a problem. I enter different things and usually find out what the medication was."

Silvia thinks it's high time doctors changed their traditional attitude about pharmacists. "They have to accept pharmacists as equal players in managing patient care," she says.

Studies have suggested that physicians are still, in many ways, stuck in the 1980s. One study of the perception of pharmacists found there was a "heavy physician dominance" in family health teams.[7] Physicians "seem to adhere to old hierarchical structures and beliefs, consistent with their professional culture," the study concluded.

"Pharmacists are still struggling for recognition," says Silvia. "Not all practitioners know what other practitioners do. My personal goal is for people to see that pharmacists are not just people behind the computers. Dispensing is part of our job. But we are also clinicians. I hope that in the future, more health care providers will recognize pharmacists as an asset."

As the number of medications increases and as the population continues to age, pharmacists will inevitably play a more important role in patient care. But the arrival of abundant, trustworthy, easy-to-access information about medications, conditions, and treatments also means that pharmacists' work, like doctors' work, is bound to change into a lifelong learning process.

It's literally impossible to remember all the new medications on the market and their possible side effects. Some side effects reappear frequently, like diarrhea and headaches; other side effects are quite rare, like a change in the sense of taste. It is critical that clinicians be able to check which adverse side effects are possible and which ones occur frequently.

As the story told by Doris, a 52-year-old pharmacist in a family health team, shows, when it comes to side effects of medications, doctors do well to draw on pharmacists' specialized knowledge and skills. Doris worked one or two days per week in a clinic in a remote rural community, and the rest of the week she worked in the pharmacy of a regional hospital.

One December morning, Doris got a call from a nurse practitioner who was part of a family health team. His patient, Duncan, a 53-year-old man who worked on a very small farm in a remote area, had been hospitalized for a blood clot in his leg. A doctor had previously put Duncan on warfarin, a commonly prescribed blood thinner. Shortly after leaving the hospital, Duncan had to go on antibiotics for a urinary tract infection.

The nurse practitioner monitored Duncan's blood using the international normalized ratio (INR), a calculation made with a blood test to determine the dose of warfarin necessary to prevent blood clots while minimizing the risk of bleeding. The INR reading said Duncan was in the right range. At first, the nurse practitioner was relieved. There didn't seem to be any negative interaction between the antibiotics and the warfarin.

The problem was that when Duncan finished the antibiotics, his blood got thicker. It was as if the warfarin stopped having an effect. "We had no idea what was going on," says Doris. "The only time he was [in the effective] therapeutic [range] was when he was on antibiotics."

Doris decided to look for the answer online. Fortunately there was no need for Duncan to come in or be examined, as he lived quite far from the clinic. Doris was pretty sure that the answer to the riddle was somewhere on the web. "I started searching in between two appointments."

Sometimes finding the right answer is a process of trial and error. This is one reason doctors sometimes hand questions about drug interactions over to pharmacists. Doris searched a number of sites. First she checked the section about drug interactions in e-Therapeutics+, then she checked Lexicomp, a widely used drug database, and Micromedics. Eventually she found a page in Lexicomp that explained exactly what she was looking for. "I learned that warfarin's anti-clotting effect is enhanced by co-trimoxazole [an antibiotic]. A low dose of warfarin was sufficient while the patient was taking co-trimoxazole but not enough once the co-trimoxazole was stopped."

In other words, Duncan was having a drug interaction that made his warfarin more effective than usual. "So when he went off the antibiotic, we had to push the dose of the blood thinner up to get the same effect."

Luckily Doris had the information she needed to convince both the doctor and the nurse taking care of Duncan. "We've had to double the dose since he left the hospital. The nurse was scared that we were going to make him bleed, and the doctor was scared that he was going to have a clot. Both needed to be, well, persuaded. We almost doubled his dose until he was in range."

Because of their specialized knowledge, pharmacists can use electronic knowledge resources to find information and come up with innovative solutions to what might seem, to doctors, like insurmountable medical problems. That was the case with Didier, a dynamic retired manager who had decided to live out his life's dream and work as a volunteer at hospitals in Africa.

Like anyone who travels or spends extended periods in tropical areas, Didier had to take an anti-malarial medication as a precaution. The question of whether to take an anti-malarial drug is one that travellers normally handle at a specialized travel clinic. However, Didier's case was complicated. He was already taking warfarin, a common anticoagulant. Naturally, he wondered if the anticoagulant would interact with the anti-malarial medication, putting him at risk. So instead of heading to a travel clinic, Didier decided to ask his family doctor.

The doctor was stumped. He was going to prescribe the anti-malarial medication Malarone (a combination of atovaquone and proguanil) but he had no idea if this could be combined with warfarin. So he decided to hand the question over to the expert: in this case, Dianna, a 31-year-old community pharmacist. The doctor asked Dianna to look for interactions between warfarin and Malarone.

The doctor couldn't have picked a more qualified professional for the job. Dianna worked part-time in a suburban family health clinic with nurses and family physicians, but she had worked with a humanitarian organization in Africa in the past. She had travelled to Africa several times to work as a volunteer in South Africa, Botswana, Zimbabwe, Zambia, and Senegal.

Dianna had also taken anti-malarial medications herself. She knew from experience that dosages had to be adapted to individual countries in Africa and even to individual regions within those countries. The risk of getting malaria also depended on the season and on the type of infection that was present in each country. In addition, the situation was changing all the time. "I asked Didier lots of questions about what areas of Africa he would be in, whether it was the rainy season, and how long he would be away for, and so we were able to gather lots of information."

Then Dianna started her search. The first thing she did was to go to the electronic version of the *Compendium of Pharmaceuticals and Specialties* (ecps), which is a comprehensive list of drug monographs published by the Canadian Pharmacists Association. "I typed in Malarone. It's a combination product so I wanted to see what the names of the two products were that were in it." Next, she went to Lexicomp and typed in warfarin and Malarone. She printed off the whole page of information that resulted from her search so that she could give it to Didier when he came in.

"What I found confirmed that warfarin therapy would have an interaction with Malarone," Dianna explained. "But how, or how much, just wasn't clear." Dianna didn't think the risks were grave enough to warrant Didier giving up his life dream of working in Africa. Instead, she came up with a strategy to help Didier find a solution then explain it to his doctor. The first step was to coordinate his two prescriptions and watch to see what happened before Didier left for Africa. Then, when Didier was actually working as a volunteer in a hospital in Africa, she would find a way to have him monitored while he was there.

"We decided to go ahead and give him the drug, but because there is a potential interaction we would monitor him frequently," Dianna explained. Dianna also proposed to Didier that he keep in touch with her by email while he was in Africa and report back to her on the results of his monitoring.

As Dianna's story shows, the arrival of abundant, trustworthy, easy-to-access information about medications, conditions, and treatments means that pharmacists' work, like doctors' work, is becoming more and more of a practice-based lifelong learning process where the "teacher" is an electronic knowledge resource combining research-based evidence and expert-based recommendations. This is very similar to the case-based learning that all professionals experience during their academic apprenticeship in nursing, pharmacy, or medicine except that in that case, the "teacher" is a senior clinical supervisor.

Dianna saw the experience as a strictly positive one. "I now know more about interactions for both malaria medications and anticoagulants. I learned what the constituents of Malarone are and how they work. In addition, I now have an understanding of how it's dosed. Because I will also do some work in Africa when I get a chance, I'll probably do more research into the antimalarial medications, too."

Easy access to trustworthy information about diseases also allows pharmacists to understand the limits of medications. One pharmacist, William, got a call from a resident who was treating Dimitri, an athletic man in his forties who was suffering from tachycardia. Most people who suffer from tachycardia are older than Dimitri and don't have symptoms. But Dimitri had palpitations, or a sense of an abnormally rapid heartbeat.

Normally, patients with tachycardia are treated with a beta-blocker. These drugs are used for high blood pressure or problems with the heart's rhythm. Dimitri had been prescribed a beta-blocker, but his tachycardia wasn't responding.

The resident wanted to know if there were other drug options before asking Didier to undergo catheter ablation, an invasive procedure used to destroy a faulty electrical pathway from the left atrium of the heart – in effect removing the direct cause of the problem. In other words, the resident was looking for a way to avoid an invasive procedure, if possible.

It was a pretty grave challenge. William set out to thoroughly examine all non-surgical possibilities for treating tachycardia. "I thought a calcium channel blocker was an option for this patient, but I had to double-check because I didn't know if that was possible for symptomatic patients," he explained. Before he could make a decision, he decided to expand his knowledge

about the condition. "I had to read up on non-medical management and to better understand the disease before I could offer
an opinion on the drug."

William searched for information in e-Therapeutics+. "I
looked for the section on pharmacologic choices, and I just
scrolled down under it to the non-pharmacologic choices." He
came to the conclusion there were no pharmacologic options
other than the beta-blocker.

"We avoided going to a higher dose that might have had
adverse effects on the patient, but not any better outcomes for
Dimitri, while he is waiting for a consultation in cardiology.
Well, we also avoided switching to a drug that didn't suit him."

In other words, knowing there is no better drug treatment
can allow clinicians to guide patients to the best course of
action, when their recommendation is backed up by trustworthy information.

Chapter 5

Better Treatment for Chronic Problems and Common Conditions

In his own way, 39-year-old Edgardo was a success story. He had been diagnosed with schizophrenia in his early twenties but had managed to live on his own until he was hospitalized six months before our story took place. Before he was hospitalized, Edgardo had spent time at a nearby family medicine clinic where he had found enough care to allow him to function outside a hospital setting.

Over the years Edgardo had established solid relationships with a group of clinicians at the clinic. He had cooperative, friendly interactions with a physician, a psychologist, social workers, and occupational therapists. When he visited the clinic, he even stopped to chat with the pharmacist who worked there part-time.

Those relationships turned out to be a great advantage when Edgardo starting having problems and was hospitalized. Like many patients suffering from mental illness, he had spent a long time finding the right treatment: side effects, like dry mouth or drowsiness, are always a challenge for patients who take anti-psychotic medication. After a long process of trial and error, his physician, Ellena, had found a medication that worked well.

Edgardo had been taking clozapine for the last seven months and his condition was stabilizing. Clozapine is often a last-resort medication for what are called treatment-resistant schizophrenia patients: patients who do not respond to other treatments. Edgardo was happy and Ellena was relieved.

Then, seven months after starting his treatment, something seemed to be going wrong. "Everything I eat and drink tastes strange," he told Ellena. "Even water tastes different."

Ellena was stumped. She had never heard of clozapine causing a change in the sense of taste. She took the problem straight to Greg, the pharmacist who worked part-time at the clinic, to see what he thought.

"It was a complicated case," Greg said, explaining that in addition to schizophrenia, Edgardo suffered from a rare condition called psychogenic polydipsia, a psychiatric condition that gives sufferers the constant feeling their mouth is dry. To treat it, Edgardo had been put on a specific diet with instructions for limited water intake. He was carefully monitored to make sure he didn't, literally, drink himself to death. "Otherwise, he would continuously drink, diluting the level of sodium in his blood, and end up having seizures," Greg explained.

Greg was also puzzled by the taste change. He was quite sure the clozapine wasn't causing it. Dry mouth is a common side effect of many medications used to treat psychiatric conditions, but to Greg's knowledge, no such adverse effect was associated with clopazine.

Ellena had another hypothesis, one she hated to admit to. She wondered if Edgardo was just trying to manipulate her into letting him change his restricted diet. "We thought maybe he was trying to get the medical team to let him eat something he wasn't allowed to eat." Before jumping to conclusions, Ellena decided to look it up.

Contrary to what many people think, medications don't come with definitive lists of side effects. There is no "bible" that tells clinicians exactly what the side effects are for any given drug.

Many side effects don't show up in clinical randomized controlled trials, in which a relatively small number of people are tested and followed up for a limited amount of time. In randomized controlled trials of drugs, the sample size can be anywhere from a few to thousands of people. There is no real standard. Trial sample sizes depend on many factors. A small sample is enough for a treatment that shows itself to be very effective in pre-trial studies, or animal studies, or pilot trials. A large sample is needed when the treatment may have low effectiveness. The duration of randomized controlled trials of drugs can also vary between days (for acute diseases), weeks, a few months (for a cancer treatment, for example), and years (for preventive interventions).

Because of this, the companies who market the drugs can't say much about what adverse effects their medication will have when it becomes available, except for effects that occur rather frequently, like nausea and headaches.[1]

Most adverse effects of medications are revealed during observational studies, which are conducted after years of drug use by millions of people. In other words, the list of side effects gets longer with time, because more is learned about drugs when they are used in the "real world." Adverse effects for specific medications are collected through reports submitted by patients and clinicians after the drug has been approved for use. Registries of adverse drug effects are built up over time, and the systems for the detection of adverse effects are quite comprehensive. In many countries, a health agency maintains an online database of information about suspected adverse drug effects. Drug manufacturers must report adverse drug effects, and health professionals and consumers can also submit reports.

There are several famous cases of drugs whose side effects did not show up in clinical trials. One is fen-phen (fenfluramine/phentermine), a drug marketed in the 1980s for weight loss. The company marketing the drug withdrew it after people who took the drug got a disease in a valve of their heart. This problem was not apparent when the US Food and Drug Administration (FDA) approved the drug.

Another famous case is, of course, thalidomide, a drug prescribed for nausea and to alleviate morning sickness during pregnancy. In the late 1950s and early 1960s, more than 10,000 children in 46 countries were born with deformities such as phocomelia (malformation of the limbs) as a consequence of thalidomide use.

In the United States, the FDA is responsible for monitoring drug safety before and after a drug receives approval for commercial distribution. Health Canada has an Adverse Reaction Database open to the public.[2] In addition, multiple printed and online monographs report drug interactions and potential adverse events. By way of illustration, the *Compendium of Pharmaceuticals and Specialties* produced by the Canadian Pharmacists Association provides more than 2,200 drug monographs that include each drug's medical indications, a description of the chemical elements of the product, dosage, warnings and precautions, drug interactions with other medications, and adverse effects. Pharmaceutical companies usually produce these monographs.

In Edgardo's case, Ellena did not want to take any chances by changing his medication. That's why she asked the clinic's pharmacist, Greg, who also knew Edgardo, for help. The stakes were high. Edgardo had tried almost every other treatment available for schizophrenia without success. "If we took him off clozapine, we knew he could just go downhill. It could lead to re-hospitalization and another cycle of chaos," Greg explained.

For a drug like clozapine that has been on the market for decades, Greg knew that a new adverse drug effect was very unlikely to pop up if it had never been mentioned before. But Greg decided to do a thorough investigation to at least eliminate the possibility that taste change had been reported as a side effect of clozapine.

Greg headed to his computer. He first looked for information on "taste disturbances with clozapine." He started by looking in UpToDate and the electronic version of the *Compendium of Pharmaceuticals and Specialties* (eCPS). "I clicked the tab 'eCPS' and then typed 'clozapine.' And then I checked Clozaril, the other name for clozapine, and looked at 'adverse effects.' I just scanned through to see if there was any report of taste changes or taste aversion or things like that. I was looking for taste change so I looked under gastrointestinal effects. And there was nothing there."

Greg then decided to look further. He did a search in MEDLINE, the database of the US National Library of Medicine, which contains millions of abstracts of research articles. "If it was a new adverse effect it was going to be reported there somewhere. I thought maybe it was a rare side effect that hadn't made it through the *Compendium of Pharmaceuticals and Specialties* yet."

Greg didn't find anything about clozapine causing taste changes in MEDLINE either. Since Greg had looked in a variety of sources and found more or less the same information, he decided, along with Ellena, to keep Edgardo on clozapine and look elsewhere to try to solve the problem.

He certainly didn't feel like double-checking was a waste of time. For one, the fact that he had done a thorough check helped him convince Edgardo to stay on his medication. "The more you explain a medication to a patient, the more he or she is likely to take it," says Greg. Most of all, it reassured him. "I was reassured because I made sure that we didn't need to take him off the medication. I was determined to make sure he stayed on clozapine. He was stable in terms of the schizophrenia," Greg explained. After thoroughly double-checking, Greg also had a clear conscience about trying an unorthodox treatment – one that turned out to be effective.

Thinking Edgardo's case over, Greg started to wonder if Edgardo's dry mouth wasn't actually a symptom of something else: the lack of variety not just in his diet but also in his life.

"Edgardo had been in the hospital for so long. It occurred to us that other things might be affecting his taste, things we weren't really thinking about."

Greg and Ellena decided to test their idea out. They would spice up Edgardo's life a bit. They arranged for an occupational therapist to take Edgardo out for lunch somewhere two or three times a week. "We still had to make sure he wouldn't drink too much, to not get sick." They also got him a television.

It seemed to work. "Edgardo's been happier because he gets out. He likes just walking to go out and eat. It's really improved his quality of life. Edgardo didn't complain about the taste change after that."

For many patients and family caregivers, watching a doctor do a double-check for medical information on the Internet might seem to make sense in the case of rare or severe health problems, but less so for chronic conditions and for patients who have been following the same treatment for some time. Those patients might wonder why their doctor is suddenly looking for information online and whether they have been getting the wrong treatment.

In fact, using electronic knowledge resources to double-check information on chronic conditions is a good idea for several reasons. To start with, in today's age of easily accessible and frequently updated medical information, it is easier than ever to verify a management plan. In the 1990s, checking for interactions between drugs was a cumbersome process that involved flipping through multiple pages, one by one. This became a daunting task when the patient took five or more medications. Today, clinicians can consult electronic knowledge resources to find information about drug interactions in just a few seconds (for two drugs) or minutes (for multiple drugs).

In most cases, when clinicians check for updates on medications and treatments, the information they find confirms that they have been doing the right thing for their patient. We did a study in 2008, examining over 2,100 searches by 40 family physicians who had looked online for clinical information. In almost half (46%) of these searches, physicians reported the information they found validated their plan. In other words, the most frequent outcome of searching for information in electronic knowledge resources was to maintain clinicians' management plans.[3]

Double-checking and refreshing memory are important aspects of medical practice. Sometimes checking improves the choice of treatment. Sometimes checking puts both doctors' and patients' doubts to rest. And sometimes doctors learn something new that will improve treatment for a patient with a similar problem in the future. Indeed, clinical information may be contradicted and revised over time. With his team, John P. Ioannidis, professor of medicine and of health research and policy at Stanford University School of Medicine, monitored citations of 49 highly cited (influential) studies that were published between 1990 and 2004 in top scientific journals. They concluded that the conclusions of seven of these studies were contradicted by the results of subsequent studies, while seven other studies "had found effects that were stronger than those of subsequent studies."[4]

Clinicians should make a habit of double-checking management plans and checking for potential drug interactions. Even though clinicians efficiently follow routines to manage common conditions, they periodically check their routines for accuracy or update and adapt them to their patients' circumstances. In addition, double-checking can help the clinician to learn something new by serendipity, a good example of learning on the job.

In the world of information studies, the expression "serendipity in information seeking" refers to a positive experience whereby a person unexpectedly finds some information that is seemingly irrelevant to their immediate goal but applies to another. For example, Roland saw a middle-aged gentleman in a walk-in clinic who complained about discomfort in one leg from previously diagnosed peripheral arterial disease, a blocked artery in his leg. As is the case with many older men, his wife had brought him in, and she did the talking. She asked Roland if he could give her husband something for his leg. "He's having trouble walking."

There are not many medical options for treating peripheral arterial disease. Roland knew of one medication that could be used (pentoxifylline), but he vaguely recalled that it wasn't effective. With a quick check of an electronic knowledge resource called DynaMed, Roland found pentoxifylline, but in the process he also saw another drug, called cilostazol, which had been shown to "increase walking distance and improve quality of life in patients" with peripheral arterial disease. This drug had been tested and had been shown to have minimal side effects. What's more, Roland learned, pentoxifylline was classified as a second-line alternative to the first choice, cilostazol. So he prescribed cilostazol.

One reason clinicians should make a habit of double-checking is that research-based evidence in the medical world can change quickly. Physicians should keep an eye out for studies that replicate and confirm or challenge the results of prior work showing the benefits of a treatment. The results of even the most highly cited randomized controlled trials might be challenged and refuted over time.

Roland has learned this on several occasions. A few years ago, one of his patients, Mary, brought her 4-year-old daughter, Anna, in for a visit. Roland knew them both very well. He had cared for Mary through a long and difficult childbirth. Anna was in excellent health except for one little problem: she had a small, stubborn *Verruca vulgaris* (otherwise known as a common wart) on her index finger.

The last time he had seen Mary about Anna's wart, Roland had advised her to try the usual treatment with salicylic acid. She had followed his instructions, but the wart hadn't disappeared. The next option was to freeze the wart with liquid nitrogen, a technique known as cryotherapy. But Roland hesitated before explaining the freezing technique to Mary. Again, he vaguely recalled reading a research synopsis (POEM) that described a simple, innovative new treatment for warts. A new study had come out showing that warts could be treated effectively with duct tape.

The Canadian Medical Association has been sending daily POEMs to Canadian physicians since 2005. POEMs are succinct descriptions of recently published research. The clinical editors choose topics for POEMs by searching the tables of contents of 102 journals for original research or systematic reviews with new information relevant to family doctors. Before writing a POEM, editors ask if patients would care about the research in question and if the research could be implemented in primary care (or if it is too specialized). They also ask if it is important enough to force changes in current practices. If it's not, then the research does not become a POEM. All POEMs conclude with a bottom-line statement that summarizes the findings of the research and helps clinicians apply the results in their practice.

Recalling the POEM that said warts could be treated with duct tape, Roland decided to look it up. The simple treatment sounded almost too good to be true. The idea of using duct tape was particularly appealing in this case because Roland knew the little girl would vigorously resist the idea of having her finger "burned" with a 10-second spray of liquid nitrogen. After a few quick taps on his smartphone, Roland located the POEM about the duct tape treatment. The short text explained exactly what the girl's mother should do: "cut the duct tape to the size of the wart and apply directly to it. Then remove it after 6 days, wash and file the wart with an emery board or pumice stone." The patient was to reapply the duct tape the next morning and to continue this cycle for two months.

Roland explained the process to Mary, who agreed to give it a try.

Unfortunately, several months later, Roland received another POEM about wart treatment, this time with a synopsis of a newer study of the duct tape approach. It turned out the duct tape option really was too good to be true. According to the newer research study, which was conducted with a better design, duct tape was no more effective in removing warts than were corn pads. In other words, duct tape was no better than a placebo.[5]

Often the initial and promising results of clinical research are subsequently contradicted. In the new age of information accessibility, this is something we all need to keep in mind.[6] In the end, Anna's wart simply disappeared. Approximately one half of children with warts are free of them after a year, even if they are not treated.[7]

We have seen many stories about doctors who found Internet-based information quickly. There are actually two ways electronic knowledge resources help doctors: they enable doctors to quickly find the information they need to diagnose or treat a particular case on the spot, and they help doctors stay abreast of new developments in the field.

No one knows this better than Dr David Slawson, professor of family medicine at the University of Virginia. Dr Slawson writes extensively about the issue of doctors finding information and keeping up to date. He travels the world speaking about what doctors need to do to find the best treatments for their patients. In the 1990s, before the Internet was even known to the broader public, he and Allen Shaughnessy (a doctor of pharmacy and an international leader in medical education) developed the concept of information mastery in medicine. Put simply, information mastery refers to the ability of doctors to use the principles of evidence-based medicine in their day-to-day practice. As we explained in chapter 1, family physicians with a general practice can see the widest possible range of symptoms and health problems. This makes it a bigger challenge for them to apply current research evidence in their daily practice. But being confronted with a myriad of conditions also makes it that much more important for family physicians to be able to find that evidence using electronic knowledge resources.

When Dr Slawson started practising, doctors were just starting to be able to get trustworthy information through these resources. Even then, Dr Slawson understood that this would change how doctors worked. In an article called "Becoming a Medical Information Master: Feeling Good About Not Knowing Everything," Drs Slawson and Shaughnessy argued that primary care clinicians could feel good about not knowing everything – and *should* feel okay about this.[8] The reason was simple. Doctors could retrieve the trustworthy information they needed by searching at the moment of need (i.e., at the point of care).

Decades later, the amount of trustworthy information available to clinicians has expanded exponentially. Unfortunately, according to Dr Slawson, not all clinicians took his advice. Today, many clinicians still do not make optimal use of the information that is readily available to them.

One problem, Dr Slawson concluded, is that medical students are still not taught how to deal with all the new information available to them. In another article Dr Slawson co-authored called "Teaching Evidence-Based Medicine: Should We Be Teaching Information Management Instead?"[9] he argued that medical schools should be teaching their students "techniques and skills to focus on finding, evaluating and using information at the point of care."

In other words, medical students should be taught specifically how to translate information they find online into better care for patients. "Every decision doctors make should be based on the highest quality information available at that time," he said in a talk at the University of Georgia.[10]

Why isn't this happening? "Busy clinicians in the real world will not look for information if they don't believe they can find it in less than a minute," Dr Slawson explains. Because many physicians don't take the time they need to find the best information, they fall back on other criteria to make their decisions. The top two forces shaping doctors' recommendations, according to Dr Slawson, are patient requests and pharmaceutical marketing.

He argues that to make good use of the information available to them, clinicians need to do two things. They need to consult what he calls "foraging" tools like newsletters and email sources. He calls these "keeping up" tools. POEMs are a good example of foraging tools. Of course, no one can possibly retain all the new information that comes out practically every day, so doctors also need what Dr Slawson calls "hunting" tools" to go out and find what they need, right when they – and their patients – need it.

Hunting tools are the electronic knowledge resources that doctors can use to get information to answer a question about a specific patient's condition or treatment. These sources filter information for relevance in a quickly accessible form at the point of care. These are the resources for clinicians to "look it up."

In pioneering work at McMaster University, Brian Haynes and his team at the Health Information Research Unit have extended the concept of the hunting tool to implement the MacPLUS Federated Search.[11] This novel approach provides a one-stop simultaneous search for evidence from multiple high-quality electronic knowledge resources such as DynaMed, for use at the point of care. Roland maintains a web portal for his practice (and residents) that is open to the public. At this portal, the reader can find links to many of the resources that we mention in this book, in a category called EBM Resources.

As we have seen, just because a medical problem is common and the treatments for it are tried and tested doesn't mean the treatments stay the same. On the contrary, medications and treatments are constantly updated as basic scientific and clinical research is carried out. That means that even in the case of very common conditions, when clinicians think they know the answers, they should be "looking it up" to make sure.

Hypercholesterolemia – high blood cholesterol – is a good example. High cholesterol affects about one in six American adults (16.2%).[12] The combination of too much "bad" cholesterol in the blood, smoking, and little physical activity dramatically increases the risk of heart attack. Diet, smoking, and a sedentary lifestyle are major risk factors for cardiovascular disease. A healthy diet and at least 30 minutes of physical activity per day help protect against heart disease. This non-medical preventive "treatment" applies to almost everyone.

However, medical treatment of high cholesterol is not as straightforward a story. As common as high cholesterol is, situations arise where clinicians need to check recommendations before prescribing medication.

This was the case for Ernie, a man in his fifties, who was already on cholesterol-lowering medication. When he saw Elizabeth, a nurse practitioner at his rural community centre, for a checkup, she noticed his cholesterol was still too high.

Elizabeth checked with Ernie's family physician and he agreed with her first instinct, which was that she should change Ernie's cholesterol-lowering medication. But there was one problem. Ernie also had a liver condition. Elizabeth suspected there might be risks in changing medication that would outweigh the benefits. So she decided to double-check her knowledge of the risks of cholesterol-lowering drugs.

Elizabeth's computer was in a separate room, so she stepped outside the examination room to perform the search. She first searched the medication Ernie was already on. She wanted to see what results they could really expect from it, to be able to evaluate the exact percentage Ernie's cholesterol might decrease. Then she decided to look it up in e-Therapeutics+.

Elizabeth learned that putting Ernie on new medication could, in fact, damage his liver. "I confirmed my hypothesis that there were some risks, and the risks outweighed the benefits. We wanted to avoid having to test him more frequently and watch him carefully." So Elizabeth and the physician ended up not changing any of Ernie's medications.

Changes in recommended dosage are one of the most common reasons doctors should double-check. When he was practising as a doctor, Pierre had a rule. With the exception of some "star" drugs like acetaminophen and penicillin, which he prescribed often, the rule was this: he would check the dosage if he had the slightest doubt about a particular medication. At the time (this was in the 1990s), Pierre checked dosages in a pocket book. And even then, maybe twice a year he got a phone call from a pharmacist who challenged his prescription.

Today, of course, it's much easier for doctors to check dosages. Roland figures that given how many thousands of drugs are available and given all the updates about them, if doctors don't check they are probably missing something, especially when it comes to side effects and interactions. Doctors who don't look up the more unusual medications they prescribe are taking a shortcut and are probably hoping the pharmacist who receives the prescription will catch something they may have missed.

In another case, 30-year-old Edmond was suffering from a general anxiety disorder. His psychiatrist had prescribed pregabalin, which is approved for use as a painkiller. In other words, he was using it off-label, meaning he was using a drug to treat a condition for which it hadn't yet been approved.

Off-label prescribing is actually quite common. Sometimes a drug is effective for a particular condition for which it hasn't been thoroughly tested. Physicians are allowed to prescribe a drug for a disease when the drug is not approved for that particular indication by a regulatory agency such as the FDA. In a nationally representative sample, Radley and collaborators examined drug-diagnosis combinations for 161 commonly used drugs and found that about 21% were used off-label.[13]

The painkiller pregabalin is used for many common conditions, and it worked well to control Edmond's anxiety. The problem was that he had had terrible constipation since he started it. He had tried everything, and nothing helped.

"He was maximized on laxative therapy, and he just couldn't handle it anymore," reported Tatiana, a young family medicine resident and enthusiastic information seeker. Constipation was a known side effect of pregabalin. A nurse asked Tatiana to stop pregabalin for Edmond. Tatiana knew there were other off-label options she could try to reduce Edmond's anxiety. The problem was switching from one medication to another. "I didn't want him to go into withdrawal. We knew he could have a serious backslide if his anxiety wasn't controlled."

Tatiana decided to propose to Edmond an anti-anxiety medication called buspirone, instead of pregabalin. She knew both medications well and was pretty sure buspirone would work for Edmond.

What she wasn't sure about was whether switching from one treatment to the other could be done simply. So she decided to double-check online. Tatiana suspected that the best solution was to progressively decrease the dose of pregabalin to avoid withdrawal adverse effects, while she started the buspirone. "There were two things I couldn't quite recall. Could I stop his pregabalin abruptly? If I had to taper it, could I give pregabalin and buspirone at the same time?" The question was all the more important since, as she put it, "pregabalin is sort of like the new big drug. I'm going to have lots of patients on it."

Tatiana first searched e-Therapeutics+ to see if pregabalin and buspirone had any interactions. She quickly checked to see if it was safe to prescribe them together, at least for a limited duration (or gradually decrease the dose of pregabalin).

Tatiana learned two things from the retrieved information: one was the tapering time for pregabalin and the other was that it had no interactions with buspirone. "I sort of happened upon the answer. But once I found it, the information was really, really, clear. It said 'taper.'"

It made sense to Tatiana. "When you start pregabalin, you increase the dose slowly, so I just worked backward." Tatiana was happy she took the time to check and confirm her hypothesis. "This search was a lifesaver. I could confidently tell Edmond that the new treatment wouldn't interact with the old one, and then I could explain to him that pregabalin had to be tapered over a week at least. I explained to him how we were going to taper it. I got his pharmacy number, and I called the pharmacy."

As we will see in the next chapter, patients also have a role to play in double-checking. Assuming that they may benefit from information to verify a plan, patients and family caregivers should simply ask their clinician whether there is a need to double-check the management plan or for potential drug interactions. It can be as simple as saying, "Is there anything that needs to be checked?"

Chapter 6

Getting Patients Engaged

Felicity was a determined 83-year-old woman who was living out her retirement in relatively good health. She only had one big problem to deal with: she suffered from osteoporosis, a common condition that causes bones to become thin and porous and increases the risk of fractures.

In fact, Felicity's real problem wasn't the osteoporosis itself. Felicity's family doctor had prescribed etidronate, a well-known medication that increases bone density. She had been taking etidronate for a while and hadn't had any side effects, but she wasn't happy with it. Taking etidronate was just too complicated for Felicity. Etidronate came in a package with a month's supply, but it wasn't as simple as just popping a pill. Every day Felicity had to swallow the tablets with a full glass of water while she was sitting. Then she had to avoid lying down for two more hours. At her age, Felicity didn't think she could keep on top of the complicated routine any longer.

Etidronate causes hypotension, or low blood pressure. People with lower blood pressure often get dizzy when they stand up quickly. That was especially risky for Felicity. If she were to fall she could easily break one of her brittle bones, an event the medication was supposed to be protecting her against.

Felicity felt there was another problem with etidronate. The medication put a damper on one of her great pleasures in life: sharing breakfast with her children and grandchildren when they visited her. Since Felicity had been instructed to take etidronate in the morning and had to wait two hours after taking it until she could eat, instead of eating breakfast with her family she had to sit and watch while everyone else ate. At her age, with her social life declining, Felicity found this frustrating.

But that wasn't even the end of it. Felicity had to take a calcium supplement along with etidronate. Was it before the etidronate or after? She could never remember.

Felicity just felt the whole thing was beyond her and wondered if there was a way to make it simpler. So she called the community health clinic she regularly visited and made an appointment with Francine, a nurse practitioner she knew.

A busy woman involved in a number of community organizations, Francine is passionate about her profession and the research she does on top of her clinical work. She understood Felicity's frustration right away and was happy to help her find a treatment that would put her mind at ease and raise her spirits.

One in three Canadian women will suffer from a fracture caused by osteoporosis during her lifetime, but osteoporosis is treatable. Francine had done some work on osteoporosis during her nursing studies and already knew a fair bit about treatment options. When Felicity came to see her, she jumped at the opportunity to broaden her knowledge further.

The main problem with Felicity taking etidronate, Francine realized, was that it involved switching back and forth between taking a pill and calcium. It was a lot to manage. Victor Montori, a professor of medicine at the Mayo Clinic and an endocrinologist (a physician who specializes in diagnosing conditions related to the glands), is well known for promoting the concept of minimally disruptive medicine (minimallydisruptivemedicine.org).

As he explained in an interview with the *Wall Street Journal*, there is pressure to make patients receive all the tests and treatments they need. But doctors, he argues, have to look at what is important to their patients and then deliver care in a way that makes sense in their context. "If you [a patient] have only one chronic condition, this is work that can probably fit into your life; but if you have multiple chronic conditions and a complex life, it is hard to fit all of this work into your day … We have to give clinicians permission to refocus on what is important for patients and deliver it in ways that fit their context … We need to deliver these treatments in a way that is mindful of the work required and the patient's capacity to get this work done."[1] Dr Montori's point was exactly what Francine was grappling with in Felicity's case. "For starters, I thought it would be easier for Felicity if she just had to take her medication once a week." Less is more.

With Felicity seated in front of her, Francine got on her computer to search for information about bisphosphonates, a family of drugs that can prevent fractures. Francine logged on to e-Therapeutics+, typed in the word "osteoporosis" and looked under "drugs used for the management of osteoporosis." Etidronate was the first bisphosphonate listed. The second was alendronate, followed by risedronate.

From her studies, Francine vaguely recalled that alendronate or risedronate could be taken once a week rather than every day. That would simplify things for Felicity. But Francine couldn't remember for sure, so she headed back to e-Therapeutics+ to see what she could find. Looking online, she discovered that both medications could be taken weekly but that alendronate had one drawback: it was known to worsen heartburn in people already suffering from it.

Francine decided to recommend Felicity try risedronate. "Easy to remember," she said. "It was taken weekly, with a calcium tablet every day."

Felicity was happy with the change and happy she'd asked Francine for an alternative. At age 83, she was not likely to start looking up information about alternative osteoporosis treatments on her own. But she didn't need to. To benefit from easily accessible online information about her disease, all she had to do was ask a clinician.

Given that Felicity had never had a fracture, another option Francine might have explored in this case was to discuss with Felicity whether she even needed to continue on her medication for fracture prevention. For conditions with no symptoms, like hypertension, many people stop their medicines too soon. For other conditions, like osteoporosis, studies have shown that continuing medicine for fracture prevention after five years provides only a very small benefit, if any at all. Knowing this, some people may choose to stop their preventive medicine for fracture prevention after five years. Others who place a higher value on the small potential for benefit may opt to continue the medicine for another five to 10 years. It's something that patients and doctors can decide together after discussing the evidence.

We've seen many ways that patients can benefit from electronic knowledge resources, and we've seen that using these resources to their fullest can lead to better quality of care for patients. The former claim is suggested by a few observational studies, including our work.[2] The latter statement is supported by experimental studies that compared the performance of clinicians with and without electronic knowledge resources (based on simulated clinical stories – no interference with real patients) and literature reviews of diverse studies conducted in everyday practice involving physician-patient and nurse-patient clinical encounters.[3] When clinicians look it up, it's not a sign they don't know what they are doing. It's a sign they are being thorough and professional.

As we've seen, clinicians can use electronic knowledge resources to double-check their diagnoses or treatments and verify information about a condition. Sometimes, they even discover information about a treatment they didn't know existed.

Online research might or might not solve a problem. But when clinicians look it up, they can always reassure patients they are doing everything they can possibly do to make sure their patients are benefitting from the most up-to-date medical information.

In this new medical universe of easily accessible information, what exactly should patients be doing? Should they be looking it up as well? Or not? When patients do look it up, should they tell their clinician what they have found?

As Felicity's story shows, health consumers don't need to be able to surf the web or sift through, analyze, and make sense of electronic knowledge resources. What they need to do is to be able to explain to their doctor, pharmacist, or nurse what's on their mind.

Roland recalls talking to physicians about a decade ago who complained about patients showing up with pages of information printed from the Internet. In this new world of online health information, the role of patients is a controversial subject, to say the least. The problem, from the doctors' perspective, was not whether patients were right or wrong about the condition they thought they had. The problem was time.

Appointment times for any doctor are limited, but even more so for family physicians. Psychiatrists may see on average one patient per hour. Family physicians will typically see four patients per hour. So when patients show up with pages of information from a medical website – Roland has faced this situation on many occasions – doctors end up spending precious time correcting patients' misunderstandings after the patients read the wrong information, or they end up having to more fully explain the information. The result is that they end up not having enough time to properly diagnose the patient's condition or agree with the patient on a treatment plan. That makes for frustrated physicians and leaves patients no further ahead.

There are still clinicians who feel uncomfortable when patients show up thinking they know what's wrong with them because they read about it on the Internet. As researchers in Montreal explained in an article published in 2014, doctors are often conflicted about the issue.[4] On one hand, "[they] recognize that Internet use allows them to explain complicated health issues more easily, and they believe Internet use has the potential to improve patient outcomes." On the other hand, "doctors are worried about Internet use exacerbating health care costs through nonessential referrals or treatments."

Things are changing. For one, doctors now realize that the Internet is just part of life. It's normal for patients and family caregivers to do their own research. The question is, how should doctors make the most of this situation?

Roland is one of the clinicians who look for ways to take advantage of the fact that patients look to the web for health information. When Roland doesn't have time during an appointment to explain a treatment in great detail, he directs patients to websites where they can learn more. This is particularly useful for patients who are either suffering from, or confronting, long-term chronic conditions or patients who require complex interventions. Roland can direct them to electronic knowledge resources that help them get their head around the choices they are facing.

On a day-to-day basis, family physicians face roughly two kinds of patients: those who require simple interventions, like taking a pill, and those who require complex interventions, like changing their diet or doing more exercise. It's certainly harder to treat a medical condition by making long-term lifestyle change than it is to treat it by taking a pill.

Michael, an old friend of Roland's, was in his late 30s when Roland got a call from Michael's wife at 6 a.m. She was in a panic. "Michael is on the floor in pain," she said. Roland drove over and took Michael to the hospital, where he had a CT scan. It turned out Michael had a kidney stone.

Though Michael recovered well, Roland knew there was more to the condition than Michael realized. Like most sufferers, Michael was unaware of the fact that kidney stones are a recurring problem. Once they've had an attack, people with kidney stones have a 70% chance of having a second or third attack.

Fortunately, there are ways to prevent further attacks, including taking medicine and changing one's diet. Diets higher in citric acid, found in citrus fruit, and lower in meat are known to help prevent kidney stones. Another option is taking a daily preventive medication, called hydrochlorothiazide, to reduce the amount of calcium in the urine.

In other words, kidney stones fall into the category of conditions requiring complex interventions. They are hard to treat, as few patients who have had a kidney stone attack are willing to make the changes they need to make to reduce the chance of future attacks. They need to be convinced.

Roland knew this, so he sent Michael to the website MedlinePlus (https://medlineplus.gov) to read about kidney stone treatments. Roland typically does this in situations when he doesn't have sufficient time to talk at length with patients.

On the website Michael would be able to read about one important and simple thing he could do to prevent future attacks: he should increase his fluid intake by drinking more water. Water dilutes the minerals (uric acid and calcium) that cause kidney stones to form.

How many of us are prepared to make lifestyle changes after a five-minute discussion with a doctor? In Roland's experience, the Internet is a useful tool for patients who require complex interventions. Reading trustworthy information from authoritative sources helps patients accept treatment. Even in the case of simple interventions, like a new prescription, some patients find it reassuring to read up about a medication they have been prescribed.

Where should patients and family caregivers go for information? Which are the best medical sites? There are no short answers to these questions (though we do provide a list of some of the most reliable sites and useful tips for searching in box 2). Focused medical subspecialists, such as orthopaedic surgeons, can refer their patients to sites specific to the types of conditions they treat. For family doctors, who treat a wide variety of

BOX 2 FINDING TRUSTWORTHY ELECTRONIC KNOWLEDGE RESOURCES – TIPS FOR PATIENTS, RELATIVES AND CAREGIVERS

1 Search high-quality consumer health information resources such as www.healthfinder.gov (US Department of Health and Human Services), https://medlineplus (US National Library of Medicine), www.mayoclinic.com, (Mayo Clinic), www.cancer.gov (US National Cancer Institute), https://familydoctor.org (American Academy of Family Physicians), and www.preventioninhand.com (College of Family Physicians of Canada).

2 Ask a librarian in your community library about high-quality electronic knowledge resources and patient organization resources; when necessary, ask a health librarian (they usually work in hospital libraries).

3 For each resource, use advanced search functions to find results on specific topics. For example, use "AND" to connect concepts, like this: "cholesterol AND diet."

4 When you find websites that look relevant, ask these questions to evaluate their credibility.

- Who are the site's sponsors? Check the web address when in doubt. For example, a government agency is indicated by .gov in the address, an educational institution by .edu, and a professional organization by .org. Commercial sites have .com in the address, and the name(s) of the sponsor(s) should be clearly identified.
- When was the website last updated? This information usually appears at the bottom of the page.
- Is the information factual? The information should include references to research articles, professional books, and specialized websites. If the information appears to be based on the authors' opinion and practice-based experience, check the expertise and credentials of the authors (authors should be qualified professionals or organizations).

5 Triangulate (compare and corroborate) information from the most trustworthy resources. If similar information appears in more than one high-quality resource, it is more likely to be credible.

6 Resources can also be found under the "patient information" category of Roland's website: http://myhq.com/public/f/a/familymedicine.

conditions, there are many sources of information that they can recommend to their patients and families. Regardless where they practise, all family physicians should have a list of their favourite sites for patient information.

A rule of thumb for patients to remember is that information can be considered to be trustworthy when similar information is found in multiple high-quality electronic knowledge resources. Patients can compare and triangulate information from several trustworthy resources, such as resources sponsored by professional organizations and patient organizations.

A rule of thumb for doctors is that they should use sites that are authoritative and not run by commercial interests. An international organization called the Health on the Net Foundation (healthonnet.org) has established comprehensive rules for reliable sites. The topics for these rules include the authority of the providers, complementarity to health care services, confidentiality, attribution of sources of information, justifiability of information, transparency, financial disclosure, and advertising distinguished from informational content.

Roland often refers his English- or Spanish-speaking patients to the website MedlinePlus (https://medlineplus.gov), which is available in English and Spanish, and his French-speaking patients to CISMeF (http://doccismef.chu-rouen.fr), which is based in Rouen, France. One great feature of MedlinePlus is interactive audio presentations about different medical conditions and treatments with slides that work like tutorials. The presentations give patients extra information doctors don't typically have time to discuss. Users can look up the side effects of a particular medication, for example, or see what other people think about it.

As mentioned in chapter 2 and illustrated in table 1, such information exchange is part of new models of doctor-patient interaction called informed decision-making and shared decision-making. The ideas are that whenever it's possible, clinicians should discuss all options with their patients. Informed decision-making should be routine: physicians recommend the best option according to the best available evidence when there is clear evidence favouring an option (e.g., when a treatment has been shown to be effective and the health benefits have been shown to outweigh the risks).

Information exchange is also the first step of shared decision-making. In this type of decision-making, the patient has to make a choice between equally acceptable options – usually, having a test or a treatment, or not. Shared decision-making can only happen when there is equipoise (no clear evidence in favour of or against a specific option in terms of benefits and risks). Clinicians can thus exchange information with their patients and engage them in a discussion about how they interpret this information on the basis of their values and preferences, which will guide the decision-making process.

Put in different terms, clinicians should be switching from the old-fashioned, paternalistic, "doctor knows best" model of medicine to a new model where clinicians take patients' concerns and preferences into account before deciding, with patients, on a preventive, diagnostic, or treatment intervention or procedure. This is particularly the case when there is some uncertainty about the effectiveness of the treatment, or the treatment is associated with significant adverse effects and small benefits. This process has been shown in numerous studies to lead to better outcomes.[5]

Trustworthy online information sources are a great tool in shared decision-making. We think both doctors and patients should embrace this model. When patients know that their doctors can find precise information quickly, they should feel all the more comfortable making their concerns known, telling their doctor what's on their mind and what they want, and asking questions. There might be a solution – literally – at their physician's fingertips.

To take advantage of electronic knowledge resources, patients don't need to be able to search for information themselves. They mostly need their doctors, nurses, and pharmacists to listen to them and then look up and share the information they need.

Fiona was a good example of a patient who intuitively understood this new model. The 55-year-old woman had been seeing her family doctor once a month to cope with insomnia, depression, and anxiety. Her psychiatrist had prescribed a benzodiazepine, a class of medication used to treat both insomnia and anxiety. Fiona was being followed by her family doctor at a family health team clinic (the equivalent of a medical home in the United States) in Ontario.

Fiona had given the benzodiazepine prescribed by her psychiatrist what she considered a fair chance, but she concluded it wasn't working. It was helping her insomnia, but not her anxiety. She asked her family doctor to see if she could find an alternative.

Unfortunately, the effectiveness of her medication wasn't the only issue Fiona was struggling with. The cost of her medication was also a burden, and worrying about that was just increasing her anxiety. Fiona wanted to find a medication that reduced her anxiety and was covered by her drug plan, the Ontario Drug Benefit Program.

When Fiona explained her concerns to her family doctor, the doctor told her about several antidepressant options that had anti-anxiety effects, but for some reason Fiona's financial preoccupations didn't seem to register with the doctor.

So Fiona took matters into her own hands. On a November afternoon, she called Frank, a pharmacist who was part of the family health team at her clinic, and explained why she wanted a new treatment to replace the benzodiazepine.

Frank understood right away. "We often use two different medications to manage depression and anxiety at the same time," Frank explained. "Since she would be taking two medications now, not just one, it was important to make sure that whatever Fiona tried was covered by her drug plan."

Frank gave Fiona a list of the medications she could take that were covered by her drug plan. "Her idea was to take the list to her next appointment so that when the doctor discussed treatments, she could check whether it was covered by her drug plan. Otherwise, there was no point wasting time talking about treatments," Frank explained.

Frank was happy to put together the list. In addition to his clinical research, he was always looking for opportunities to broaden his knowledge. Frank went straight to e-Therapeutics+ and looked up anti-depressants that were also used to treat anxiety. "I went into 'psychiatric disorders' and then into 'anxiety disorders' and then 'pharmacologic choices' and that's where they were."

Frank printed the table of possible treatments, put a little check mark beside the ones that were covered by the Ontario Drug Benefit Program, and faxed the list to the doctor.

Fiona returned to see her doctor to talk about the list. To her astonishment, her doctor ignored it – or at least that was the only explanation she could come up with. "The doctor told her that she had received the list, but then she went ahead and prescribed something that wasn't covered," said Frank.

Fiona didn't give up, and neither did Frank. Fiona's doctor had announced she was leaving the office the following week for a month of vacation, so the clock was ticking, and Fiona needed a solution. When he heard this, Frank called the doctor right away. "Your patient has no medication. We need to resolve this issue," he explained. "If we don't deal with this today, Fiona will have no medication for a month. You need to get hold of the psychiatrist and have a discussion with her and get this changed to something that's appropriate."

Fiona's family physician finally got the message. The following Monday, she called Frank back. "Fiona came back to me with another prescription and the problem was solved," said Frank.

Chapter 7

The Pros and Cons of "Doctor Google"

In 2010, 80% of Canadian households were connected to the Internet.[1] In the United States, 87% (99% of 18- to 29-year-olds) were connected in 2015.[2] The Internet is now the most frequently accessed platform for finding consumer health information.[3] Access to other sources of health information has decreased.

Almost everybody uses online health information, either directly or mediated by someone else, such as a relative, a librarian, or a professional. For example, a 2015 survey of a representative sample of 23,693 parents of preschool children in Quebec showed that only 1.5% of parents never know where to find information on children.[4] There may be several reasons why these rare "information poor" individuals don't use information: they may perceive themselves as people who cannot be helped, they may be secretive and mistrust others, and they may consider exposure to information as a risk (with the harm outweighing benefits).[5] Typically, they have a low literacy level and have few or no communication skills or social networks to help them overcome their literacy barrier (e.g., they may face severe mental health issues, or they may live outside the contemporary information society for religious reasons).

As the years go by, we believe clinicians will have to get used to the fact that almost all patients look online for health information by themselves. Use of the Internet has become routine, but the phenomenon of patients using online information to "self-diagnose" still provokes mixed reactions from doctors, nurses, and pharmacists.

The Pew Research Center, which is based in Washington, DC, compiled the results of multiple nationwide surveys of Americans to assess how individuals were using the Internet to find health and medical information.[2] Not surprisingly, the most frequent seekers of online health information are young, affluent (with household incomes of $75,000 or more), and educated (with one or more college degrees). Women are more likely than men to look online for health information.

At the same time, the Pew Research Center looked into *how* people looked online for health information. Rather than looking up information in targeted, reliable online consumer health information resources, like the ones discussed in the previous chapter, over three-quarters (77%) of Internet health information seekers started by typing keywords into Google or another search engine. Only 13% of those surveyed said they consulted a site that specialized in health information, like MedlinePlus. A very small minority, 2%, went to a general site like Wikipedia for information. An even smaller percentage (1%) looked for information via a social network site, like Facebook. Interestingly, one adult in three (35%) in the United States reported they looked online to try to "figure out the medical condition they or another may have." The Pew researchers called this group online diagnosers.

This news shouldn't be too alarming for health professionals. Despite the spike in Internet use for finding health information, the Pew Research Center found that most people still trust doctors over other sources of information. According to the surveys, when looking for health information, care, or support, 70% of US adults first go to a doctor or to another health care professional.

However, doctors still tend to be somewhat defensive when it comes to patients looking information up on their own. One reason is that some clinicians believe that looking randomly online just increases people's anxiety about their health, rather than helping them to get better treatment. A new term, "cyberchondria," has popped up in recent decades as a label for this phenomenon.

According to the *Journal of Neurology, Neurosurgery, and Psychiatry*, the term cyberchondria first appeared in a 2001 article in the UK daily the *Independent*, to describe "the excessive use of internet health sites to fuel health anxiety." Cyberchondria has been defined as "the unfounded escalation of concerns about common symptomology based on a review of search results and literature online."[6] In other words, when someone thinks a headache means they have a brain tumour, on the basis of what they've read online, they are suffering from cyberchondria.

No scientific study has conclusively shown whether going online to search for health information increases people's anxiety about their health or decreases it. The study that came closest was conducted by a pair of Microsoft researchers in the United States, Ryen White and Eric Horvitz.[7] Unfortunately, their study results cannot be generalized. The number of people who responded to the survey was small (about 500 people) and the participants were all Microsoft employees, who are hardly representative of the general population. The response rate was also very low (10%), so the authors cannot really conclude anything about the behaviour of Microsoft employees because most of them did not answer the survey.

Still, what they found is thought provoking. White and Horvitz tried to determine whether the web was actually creating unwarranted concerns over health, so they simply asked the people who completed their survey, "Do Web searches make you more worried about your health? Or do they reassure you?" Interactions with the web increased medical anxiety for about two of every five respondents. Almost one-half of the individuals who responded to their questionnaire claimed using the web actually *reduced* their anxiety about a health matter.

A few years later, the researchers set out to explore whether online health information searches, by their very nature, contributed to the spread of cyberchondria. In other words, was there was something about the Internet itself that made users think common symptoms (like headaches or fatigue) were signs of a serious disease? The researchers referred to this effect as "escalating" medical concerns.

The researchers found there was an escalating effect but only for a minority of people, about one in five. They explained, "The Web has the potential to increase the anxieties of people who have little or no medical training, especially when a Web search is employed as a diagnostic procedure."

What the study really suggests, in our view, is that people who are already anxious about their health, people who are prone to self-diagnose, might indeed become more anxious when they do Google searches about their symptoms. This also might be more likely to happen with individuals who aren't familiar with how web pages are ranked on search engines like Google.

White and Horvitz concluded that part of the escalation of medical concerns had to do with the way people were looking for information. Starting to search for medical information with a search engine like Google, they say, was not a good idea.

The problem is that people have no idea how search engines work. Three in four of their respondents reported that they thought the ranking of web search results indicated the likelihood of the illness. In other words, they assumed that the pages that came up first in their search results were the most authoritative or that the conditions that came up first were the most likely diagnoses for their symptoms.

In fact, that's not the way search engines like Google currently work. As White and Horvitz put it, web search engines "are not designed to perform coherent diagnostic reasoning, which would require probabilistic reasoning methods." Search engines rank sites according to both the number of visits the sites get (a measure of their popularity) and their number of links to other pages (a rough measure of their authority).

The nature of the web itself may also skew results in a way that's bound to make people more worried. As the researchers point out, there is more written on the web about serious conditions than common conditions: "headaches are far more often caused by caffeine withdrawal than by cerebral hemorrhage or brain tumours, but there is a great deal written about the link between headaches and the more serious, albeit rare ailments." So in some ways the Internet, by its very nature, leads people to think they have a more serious disease than they probably do (like when you type in "headache" and come up with information on brain tumours).

By opening pages about the most serious conditions, the cyberchondriacs who consult the web frequently push those pages to the top of the ranking in search engines in a self-perpetuating cycle of misinformation. The authors conclude, "If the worried well are more drawn to content about potentially serious concerns than about more likely (but less worrisome) explanations, the ranking of web pages on rare but serious disorders could be skewed towards the top of ranked lists." Information scientists and computer scientists are aware of these issues, and things may change in the near future when the results of international multicentre research programs such as Clef eHealth (https://sites.google.com/site/clefehealth2016) are incorporated into search engines.

It's quite a different story when patients and family caregivers consult trustworthy, reliable electronic knowledge resources targeting general consumers, especially the ones that we have suggested (or that any clinician can suggest). We have read and analyzed a great number of studies on the topic. Most of these studies conclude that people generally become *less* anxious about their health when they consult trustworthy electronic knowledge resources, as long as they know these are trustworthy resources.

Multiple studies show that when patients find and use online information they are more satisfied overall with all aspects of health care: they participate more in health decision-making, they are more engaged in their health care, and they experience more health benefits. In other words, when people consult trustworthy information recommended by a clinician, they feel they get better care, and that helps them feel better.

For example, in 2014–15 we conducted a longitudinal survey to evaluate the user's viewpoint on the value of a reliable, free online resource that provides parenting information to new parents and parents with young children (naitreetgrandir. com).[8] This resource includes a website and newsletter that provides free, independent, and trustworthy information to equip parents and families (e.g., grandparents) during pregnancy and the first eight years of their children's lives (it is funded by the philanthropic Lucie and André Chagnon Foundation). Many clinicians direct their patients to this popular resource (about 75% of parents of preschool-aged children use this website in Quebec). We received 17,545 responses to our survey that assessed information from specific web pages between 1 June 2014 and 31 January 2015. Roughly four out of five parents (72%) said they thought the information would benefit themselves or their child. Among the top expected benefits: one-third of respondents (35%) said the site's information helped them "worry less." Only 48 respondents (0.3%) suggested that using information from the website might harm their child's health (e.g., "information may be unclear and cannot replace professional advice") or their own health (e.g., "increase parents' guilt when unhealthy behaviours are pursued such as smoking").

In addition, 2,437 respondents completed a demographic questionnaire, which allowed us to compare the responses from respondents who had a low level of education and a low level of income with the responses of other respondents (who had a higher level of education or income). Low-education, low-income participants were more likely than the other participants to seek and use information from the website for the children of others (relatives, friends, and other members of their social network), to be more engaged in decision-making for their child after reading information on the website, and to be less worried about a problem concerning their child after reading information on the website (statistically significant differences; p value < 0.01). This suggests that trustworthy, high-quality online parenting information with audio content on each page may be particularly beneficial for vulnerable parents.

In 2013, Pierre, along with 12 other health professionals, analyzed in-depth interviews with 16 health consumers (lay people who had no training or experience in health sciences or information studies) to gather their impressions of the pros and cons of using online health information. All 16 interviewees could read and interpret most health texts, what we would call moderate health literacy. All of them reported that they frequently searched for health information on the Internet.[9]

In this set of interviews, Pierre and his collaborators also found that not all experiences with online health information are positive. One respondent described the Internet as a double-edged sword. Another reported, "The more information I have, the more I will worry." Another said, "Maybe it's too much information, but I'd rather know more." One interviewee commented on the "dangers" associated with looking up symptoms: "You put in how you feel and it will tell you [you] have cancer, you have gout, you have arthritis … You've got every single disease in the world."

More interestingly, their work unveiled a worrisome trend. Interviewees were asked whether they used online information in a discussion with a health professional. Almost unanimously, the interviewees said that they never discussed the information they found online with their health professional. In other words, the problem is not that people search, but that they are too afraid or too intimidated to talk to their doctor about what they find.

One described the situation like this: "A lot of doctors don't like their patients to come up with information. They really dislike it; it's their domain." Another interviewee shared a similar opinion: "You have to be quite careful [about] saying 'I have been reading on the Internet, and this could be that or maybe we should look at that treatment'; [the doctor] is not very open to his patients playing doctor."

This reluctance to discuss online health information with health professionals is commonly reported in information studies, and it represents a big barrier to informed decision-making and shared decision-making. How can patients be more engaged in their care when they hesitate to share and use the information they find? Sharing information seems to generally happen only in one direction (from clinicians to patients); our work may facilitate the two-way exchange of knowledge (from patients to clinicians and from clinicians to patients).

Researchers from McGill University wrote, "When it comes to confirming online health-related information with their physicians, many patients are hesitant; some patients are afraid their doctors might perceive it as a challenge to their expertise and authority, highlighting the need for open dialogue between doctors and patients about online health information and appropriate electronic knowledge resources."[10]

So what should patients do if they want to exchange information they have found? They should ask their nurses, pharmacists, and physicians to recommend a trustworthy online resource that they can use to increase their knowledge about and engagement in their own health care, namely a resource complementary to and possibly better than the one(s) they already searched. In the same vein, what should doctors do if they want to make the most of the fact that patients look for health-related information online? The first step is to express their openness to it. For patients, searching online is an activity they routinely undertake. Doctors have to accept this, if they haven't already.

We have been discussing how to prevent patients and families from getting incorrect health information. Therefore, it's fair to wonder how often clinicians get the wrong answer even if they are using a reliable online information source. We decided to explore this question. We found six studies that suggest that a search for information to answer a clinical question can lead a clinician to change a correct answer to an incorrect answer.[11] All six studies used simulated clinical stories – in other words, they did not interfere with real patients or clinical encounters – and five of them were actually conducted in computer laboratories. The most important finding was that after clinicians searched for information, more incorrect answers became correct than vice versa. Aside from these six studies, we found no research that reported any adverse events associated with information seeking (patients getting worse, rather than better) in primary care, although this obviously happens in real life. Nevertheless, all the studies suggested that overall, the effect of a clinician doing an active information search was positive for patients.

Doctors have a choice: they can either react defensively, and in the process risk dismissing their patients' true concerns, or they can discuss the information their patients or their patients' family members have brought to them with the patient and family caregivers, if for no other reason than to better understand what's on their mind and to discuss trustworthy information from high-quality online consumer health information resources. If doctors choose the latter option, it will go a long way toward improving care.

We have seen that when patients talk to clinicians about their concerns, they get simpler and cheaper care thanks to online searches. In some situations, talking openly about a problem can even prevent a patient from abandoning treatment altogether.

This was the case for Freddy, a 65-year-old man who had been on medication for benign prostatic hyperplasia, a benign enlargement of the prostate that restricts the flow of urine.

Freddy was taking tamsulosin, which relaxes muscles near the bladder so urine can flow more easily.

After he began his treatment, Freddy started experiencing a rather embarrassing side effect: priapism, a sustained erection. He had done his research and already knew there was an alternative medication for his condition, called finasteride. But he wondered if the alternative would give him the same problem.

After some hesitation, Freddy decided to open up about his problem to a clinician. He made an appointment with Vanessa, a 31-year-old community pharmacist who works part-time in a suburban family health team. Freddy asked Vanessa if tamsulosin was causing the side effect and whether switching to finasteride would help or just do the same thing.

"I looked at whether priapism can be caused by Freddy's medication," Vanessa reported. "I checked on each drug in the ecps [the electronic version of the *Compendium of Pharmaceuticals and Specialties*]. I scrolled down and read everything as I went. I skimmed through the 'warnings and precautions' to see if there was anything in there and then looked at the 'adverse drug reactions' where there were two paragraphs. I looked at a section called 'action in clinical pharmacology' for both of them just to see how they act, to see if there wouldn't be anything that would tend to make one more inclined to cause that side effect than the other."

Vanessa's conclusion was that Freddy would probably be better off switching to finasteride, as he thought. "So I explained to him how the drug worked, and then he made the decision with me to switch."

In the end, Vanessa felt her search had more than solved Freddy's problem. It had kept him on medication for his condition. "He felt assured that switching was an okay thing to do. I think if he hadn't talked to me about his problem, he might have stopped taking the drug altogether."

Chapter 8

Nurses and Doctors Can't Remember Everything

Henry and his mother really didn't need any more problems. Henry was 37 years old, mentally challenged, and living at home with his parents. His family doctor had recently diagnosed him with diabetes. The doctor thought Henry had probably gone undiagnosed for quite some time.

Henry's doctor prescribed metformin for him. Metformin is an oral medication that stimulates the body's production of insulin, which meant Henry didn't need to start injecting insulin. Henry's latest blood tests showed that the level of glucose in his blood was lower than before. In other words, he was reacting well to the medication.

Then, suddenly, one October morning, a cloud appeared on the horizon. Henry was at a clinic in his small town. He was sitting with Roxanne, a nurse practitioner, who was checking the results of his last round of blood tests. Roxanne noticed that Henry's creatinine levels were increasing.

Creatinine is a substance eliminated by the kidney as they flush waste out of the bloodstream. When the level of creatinine increases, it's usually a sign of kidney trouble. "We had no idea what was going on," said Roxanne.

Roxanne couldn't remember many details about metformin on the spot, but she did recall that guidelines for metformin use recommended that doctors not prescribe it to patients with kidney failure. She also recalled that metformin was known to cause lactic acidosis, or a low level of blood pH, which is another sign of kidney malfunction. Roxanne knew that severe acidosis – when the kidneys cannot normalize pH levels – can lead to coma or even death.

In other words, Roxanne knew Henry's problem could become really serious and might require immediate attention. The safest and fastest solution, she knew, was to take him off metformin. Before making a decision, though, she thought she should check the facts about metformin and kidney malfunction. Had Roxanne been working 20 years ago, before anyone could quickly find information about specific situations like Henry's on the Internet, she might have had to forego investigating and just act quickly. As it was, she went online to see what she could find. "I wanted to know what was the cut-off point, when you should stop taking the metformin. I knew there were limits, but I couldn't remember what they were."

Henry's case was special. He had been diagnosed with diabetes very late in the progression of the condition. "He'd probably had diabetes for a long time," Roxanne said. Since his medication was working, she felt that his late diagnosis made it all the more important to keep him on the treatment. "At the very least, if we did need to change his medication, I wanted to be able to explain why."

So Roxanne logged onto e-Therapeutics+. On that site she could access the eCPS, the electronic version of the *Compendium of Pharmaceuticals and Specialties*, which is the Canadian reference for drug information. Created in 1960, it is maintained by the Canadian Pharmacists Association to provide up-to-date information about medications: what ingredients or chemical they consist of, how to use them, how to store them, and more. All doctors have access to the printed CPS, but the ECPS is infinitely easier to use than the traditional book version.

Roxanne didn't find what she was looking for with a quick search. So she turned to one of the doctors at her clinic to see if he had any suggestions. The doctor sent her back to her computer and suggested she log on to the website of the Canadian Diabetes Association. There, Roxanne found information that confirmed what she had suspected: by taking metformin, Henry could end up in a vicious circle. Metformin can on rare occasions cause kidney malfunction, which in turn can provoke lactic acidosis (among other things), which in turn causes kidney malfunction.

Although Henry's level of creatinine had increased, Roxanne discovered that it was still within the safe range. Creatinine levels, she learned, can be a little higher than normal without cause for concern as long as they are stable and not increasing. When the level rises beyond the safe range, patients might need to be hospitalized or, eventually, have dialysis.

Roxanne's information search reassured everyone: Henry, his mom, and their family physician. "I was relieved. I really didn't want to change the medication he was taking. The site provided detailed guidelines on what range of creatinine was safe for someone taking metformin."

Clinicians can't remember everything. It's simply impossible to retain all the pieces of medical information out there.

In the International Classification of Diseases (ICD), compiled by the World Health Organization, there are about 15,000 codes for diseases, organized into 15 categories.

The use of information is one of the biggest differences between clinicians with specialized practice and clinicians with general practice. For instance, a physician with a specialized practice may use knowledge and information on about 1,000 ICD codes, on average. A physician with a general practice, on the other hand, is more likely to use knowledge and information from all 15,000 codes in the ICD. Of course, specialists sometimes also look for information about diseases from outside their speciality.

The range and complexity of information that family physicians with a general practice have to deal with can make their day-to-day work very challenging. Handling complex information is a significant part of their work, but it is not necessarily a drawback. For instance, we were drawn to this field, like many other primary care clinicians, because we seek variety. Information searches are part of our job, and we enjoy carrying them out.

But not all clinicians are comfortable with the idea of searching for and verifying information on a regular basis. Many family physicians look for ways to reduce the amount of information they need to master, and they often turn to one solution: they focus their practice, say, on maternity care or care of the elderly. Because of this trend, some predict that true generalists may become rare in the 21st century.

Indeed, family physicians who don't have focused practices are now a minority, albeit a large one. In 2007, the ratio of family physicians with a specialized practice compared with those with a general practice, also called womb-to-tomb practitioners, was roughly 50-50. Eight years later, in 2013, in a National Physician Survey of over 60,000 Canadian family physicians, only two out of five family physicians (38.2%) reported their practice was truly general. A full 62% of respondents specialized in one clinical area.

Again, one reason family physicians opt to focus their practice is that it reduces the amount of information they need to recall, or look up, in their everyday work. Finding information is even more challenging for doctors who work, say, in a rural clinic, where they don't have access to specialists as they would in an urban setting.

Doctors do forget, especially given the fact that patients can arrive at their office with almost any imaginable medical condition. But doctors aren't the only ones who forget. As Hazel, a 42-year-old family physician, discovered, doctors sometimes have to look things up because patients have forgotten to provide an important piece of information.

Hazel worked in a suburban primary care clinic and part-time at the emergency department of her local hospital. She had just returned to work after a vacation when George, a 65-year-old, came into the emergency department complaining of chest pain.

George described his pain to Hazel. She then asked him a series of questions to get his medical history. This is standard practice for doctors, and it helps them identify or eliminate possible diagnoses.

George told Hazel he had recently been diagnosed with diabetes. It was evidently on his mind. As Hazel continued down the list of standard questions, she asked him if he had previously had any heart problems. To her amazement, George revealed that he had a cardiac defibrillator, a small device implanted in his chest to help treat an irregular heartbeat. "It was like he'd just remembered."

Hazel couldn't believe her ears. This kind of information would normally have been the first thing a heart patient told her. "He said he didn't even know why he had it. I thought, well, he may have had cardiac arrest in the past. Maybe he was given the information when he was in bad shape and just didn't remember."

Hazel was all the more troubled because she had forgotten some of what she had learned about cardiac defibrillators. "I'm very familiar with the antiarrhythmic drugs for the heart (cardiac drugs), and I'd learned about defibrillators, but since I had never treated anyone with one of these implanted devices, I'd sort of forgotten," she admitted.

In particular, Hazel had forgotten what the treatment plan was for patients with cardiac defibrillators. "It was kind of one of those moments when you say, 'Wait a minute,' like a trigger in your brain." Hazel was pretty sure George should be having regular follow-up with a cardiologist. She headed to her computer to see what she could find. She first checked on e-Therapeutics+. Scanning through the information on cardiac defibrillators, Hazel also updated her knowledge, reading the latest information about their effectiveness for controlling an irregular heartbeat.

While reading the online information, Hazel confirmed at least one thing she suspected, namely that cardiac defibrillators required complex evaluation and follow-up. That gave her all the information she needed to convince George it was important to see a cardiologist. "I told him there's a 39% reduction in mortality after a year with a cardiac defibrillator, compared to the use of medication. So I could reassure him it was really helping. Then I explained that because of the complexity of the device, he really needed to be seeing a specialist on an ongoing basis, for follow-up."

George got the message. He returned to his family doctor the next week to discuss it. The doctor recommended the same thing as Hazel. "After two recommendations in two weeks, he finally connected with his cardiologist," Hazel said.

Do old doctors forget more than young doctors? Maybe, but that's not the problem. When it comes to searching for information, the medical world has something of a generation gap. Patients should be aware of it.

The median age of doctors is 45. That puts the medical field in a situation where half of clinicians were trained in the pre-Internet era and the other half in the post-Internet era. Anyone over 45 (at the time we wrote this book) was trained in the 1980s or earlier and is considered to be a "digital immigrant." Anyone trained from the 1990s on is considered a "digital native."

Roland teaches evidence-based medicine and information mastery techniques to medical students and residents. As digital natives, most young doctors today are used to looking for information online, on the spot. For them, the idea of integrating information searches into their regular decision-making is usually a no-brainer.

The generation gap really shows up when young doctors start working in hospitals and clinics. They just assume their older colleagues are as comfortable "looking it up" as they are, so they are sometimes in for a shock: what they often see in the real life of medical practice is that old doctors make decisions without looking anything up.

Older doctors are sceptical when they see younger colleagues "with their noses in their phones all the time." The older doctors think their younger colleagues are wasting time on their mobile devices, perhaps even looking at Facebook. Some older doctors consider this a sign of deviant behaviour. Even when the younger doctors find important medical information on a mobile device, some older doctors see it as a threat, as if the younger doctor is challenging their judgment.

This generation gap will disappear as today's young doctors make room for the even more technologically savvy junior doctors coming up. In the meantime, though, another problem keeps doctors from "looking it up." It's called the shortcut.

When Roland teaches young doctors the principles of evidence-based medicine and how to use electronic knowledge resources (information mastery), he begins the class by telling the doctors that when they have a clinical question, they have four choices:

1 Refer the patient to a specialist.
2 Have an informal discussion with an expert.
3 Find the answer yourself (use a knowledge resource).
4 Ignore the question.

As the last choice is not good for patient care, and experts are not always around, the choice boils down to two options. Doctors can search for trustworthy information to answer their question, or they can refer the patient to a specialist.

In 2001, two British ethnographers, John Gabbay and Andrée le May, studied how family physicians actually "looked it up" before making decisions about a diagnosis or treatment.[1] The two researchers were curious about how doctors first stop to think about whether they know something or not and eventually search for information to either answer their question or confirm what they thought.

Gabbay and le May decided to take a close look at decision-making in two different practices, one rural and one urban. Lawndale was the alias they used for a rural teaching practice in the south of England where the population is relatively elderly and middle class. Urbchester was the alias they gave to an inner-city practice in the north of England that treats a high proportion of unemployed and immigrant patients as well as students.

The pair found that doctors rarely "looked it up" in their day-to-day work. As they explained, "individual practitioners did not go through the steps that are traditionally associated with the linear-rational model of evidence-based health care – not *once* the whole time they were observing them." As the researchers noted, the doctors in the study didn't look at clinical guidelines either, in paper form or electronically. They did, however, point to laminated guidelines on their walls when they were explaining something to a patient.

The researchers concluded, "Clinicians rarely accessed and used explicit evidence from research or other sources directly." Instead, they relied on what the researchers called mindlines, or collectively reinforced, internalized, tacit guidelines acquired over years of experience treating specific conditions. As the researchers explained, "These [mindlines] were informed by brief reading but mainly by their own and their colleagues' experiences, their interactions with each other and with opinion leaders, patients, and pharmaceutical representatives, and other sources of largely tacit knowledge."

Gabbay and le May noted that "although the practice's sophisticated computer system allowed easy direct access to several accepted expert systems, and more generally to the internet, family physicians very rarely used them." The doctors they studied estimated that they used computers to look things up "less than once every week; even then it would probably be only to download information to give to patients," and the researchers said that "we never saw them use such systems to solve a clinical problem in real time."

There were limits to this research, which Gabbay and le May acknowledged. Their findings were based on information from only two clinics in the United Kingdom, each with its own particular culture. The researchers did know of practices where doctors made better and more frequent use of online information. Still, the two practices they studied were acknowledged to be "among the best in their localities."

Roland calls this tendency to take shortcuts a choice between "think" and "blink." The idea came from two important books on decision-making. The journalist and essayist Malcolm Gladwell argues that decisions made on instinct are often as good as ones made by consulting volumes of research. The former can be called blink decisions, and everyone makes them, including doctors. In his 2011 book *Thinking, Fast and Slow*, Nobel laureate Daniel Kahneman describes blink thinking, which he calls system 1 thinking, as "mental shortcuts that usually involve focusing on one aspect of a complex problem and ignoring others."[2] System 1 thinking, he explains, "operates automatically and quickly, with little or no effort and no sense of voluntary control." In contrast, system 2 thinking "allocates attention to the effortful mental activities that demand it, including complex computations."

Blink thinking is not all bad. Judging a situation quickly does not necessarily mean you will come to the wrong conclusion. People do it all the time, and sometimes they have no choice. It's a normal part of how we think. But on the whole, Roland thinks doctors, nurse practitioners, and pharmacists would do better not to rely too heavily on blink thinking. There are risks to it. As Kahneman argues, system 1 (blink) thinking, or the "spontaneous search for an intuitive solution," sometimes fails.

System 1 thinking is attractive for more reasons than the fact that it is fast. The world values overconfidence, Kahneman argues, and system 1 thinking projects an image of confidence: it makes people look like they know the answers. This phenomenon is particularly true for doctors, and it is one reason doctors are more apt to give a diagnosis right away than admit they should think it over.

"Acting on pretended knowledge is often the preferred solution," Kahneman writes. "Confidence is valued over uncertainty and there is a prevailing censure against disclosing uncertainty to patients."

In other words, even though doctors don't know everything – and no one should expect them to – patients tend to want to believe they do. Doctors themselves have to face this problem. The reality is that, more often than not, doctors take shortcuts to make decisions instead of looking things up. It's not that doctors are lazy. They just tend to act on what they know – or, actually, what they *think* they know. In other words, a lot of doctors don't know what they don't know.

Luckily, things are changing, though perhaps not quickly enough. More and more physicians are getting comfortable "looking it up" and being alerted to new knowledge through the daily POEMS and weekly Highlights we mentioned earlier, for instance. Over the course of our research, we have met many clinicians who make system 2 thinking part of their everyday work, who "look it up" on a regular basis. As Roxanne, the nurse practitioner we introduced above, told us, "I love the little bits of information I receive from POEMS and other highlights of research. Nurses don't receive regular information updates as often as doctors. For one, pharmaceutical companies are less likely to come into our offices and explain their products. Nurses get almost no new information about treatments unless we seek it out. So it's great to receive things electronically."

Medicine is a changing field, and doctors *need* to change their habits more than ever. They can't afford to keep doing things the way they did.

In fact, all doctors today are expected to update their knowledge and learn about new research and knowledge in their field. This is known as continuing medical education. Not all doctors are especially enthusiastic about doing continuing education and some get complacent about keeping up to date. They think, "I'm too busy," or "I'm good enough," or "I have other things to do."

But that is changing. For one, many jurisdictions have decided to make continuing education mandatory. Doctors now have to report their educational activities on an annual basis. Canadian family physicians, for example, have to submit proof of 250 continuing education credits per five-year period or risk losing their membership in the College of Family Physicians of Canada.

In some ways, continuing medical education is a bigger challenge for family physicians with a general practice than it is for physicians with a specialized practice, mostly because generalists have to choose what new medical developments to follow. A specialist can go once a year to the conference for her specialty and has one or two specialized journals to read on a regular basis. In contrast, a generalist would have to go to every medical conference and read all of the medical journals to truly stay up to date on advances in his field. Of course, that's simply not possible, which is why electronic knowledge resources can help clinicians in family medicine do their job better than ever. We met one doctor who told us a story of how he understood what he didn't know and how turning to these resources helped him fill in knowledge gaps.

Grant, an experienced 57-year-old family doctor, works in the family health clinic of an academic hospital. He combines clinical practice, research, and teaching of medical students and residents. He is enthusiastic about using technology in his practice and even created a website for his clinic, which includes a list of links to trustworthy educational materials for patients, family caregivers, students, and residents.

When we met him he wanted to talk about a recent patient, a newborn baby named Gabriella. Gabriella's parents brought her to the clinic in a panic. She was clearly jaundiced. The first thing Grant did was tell them to relax while he did a quick information search to find out whether Gabriella's jaundice was dangerous. "My initial management plan was to send the baby to a lab for a blood test. Then I realized I should answer that question first."

Grant decided to consult a clinical decision support system. Decision support systems are computerized checklists and calculators designed to help physicians make more informed decisions.[3] They are based on unambiguous algorithms and programmed to provide physicians with specific procedures for solving well-known problems in simple situations. For example, a typical algorithm might be as follows: "*Patients with symptom A and symptom B need an X-ray. Patients do not need an X-ray when they have symptom A alone, or symptom B alone, or neither symptom A nor symptom B.*" Some decision support systems provide a checklist of symptoms or findings on physical examination. After checking the symptoms that apply, physicians get a recommendation, like "*do an X-ray*" or "*do not do an X-ray.*"

Decision support systems are based on thorough research. Using them allows physicians to get solutions without reading the lengthy documents used to create the algorithms. They save time and prevent errors, but they only address a small minority of clinical situations.

Neonatal jaundice is one of the situations covered by decision support systems. Grant knew he needed a way to quickly assess Gabriella's situation. "I saw Gabriella four days after she was born, and jaundice at that time may become dangerous." He went online to Essential Evidence Plus and found exactly what he was looking for: a decision support system for jaundice. Grant then entered specific data about this baby and obtained a recommendation.

Using the tool, Grant saw that Gabriella really was in danger. "I changed my plan from 'send her for blood tests' to 'send her to the hospital.' I told the parents to take her to a hospital right away."

Clinical decision support systems can also help prevent drug interactions by using algorithms that analyze data on drug prescriptions from health administrative databases.[4]

We met Geneviève, a calm 31-year-old in the second year of her family medicine residency. In her work, she carries a tablet around with her all the time so she can look up information whenever she feels the need. At the time, she was following about 150 patients (she called them "her" patients). She had her own list of favourite electronic knowledge resources, including e-Therapeutics+, which she said provided "useful and accurate information."

Geneviève was in the emergency department of the hospital when Hudson, a man in his 60s, arrived complaining of chest pain. She considered prescribing nitrates, which are commonly used to relieve pain in patients with angina. But she decided to look for information first. "I was afraid he was having a heart attack."

Geneviève said she was just "reviewing the information" about angina on e-Therapeutics+ when she came across something that made her stop in her tracks. "I was just going through the whole article, just to refresh my memory. Then I saw some information I had forgotten: that nitrates interact with other drugs, including sildenafil [sold as Viagra]." Given Hudson's age, Geneviève thought it might be a good idea to double check with the patient to see if he happened to be taking sildenafil.

"I already knew about sidenafil. It's not something that I routinely ask patients, it's just that I saw a little green Highlight on nitrates, and it just sort of jogged my memory." Because of the retrieved information, the resident remembered "that nitrates combined with drugs such as sildenafil cause a sudden drop in blood pressure, which can, you know, in certain conditions, kill the patient."

It was a good thing Geneviève checked. As it turned out, Hudson had taken sildenafil less than 24 hours earlier. So Geneviève looked for a safe alternative. "Hudson was on nitrates, but he was on other cardiac medications as well. So I kept the other medications and stopped the nitrates."

While information provided by patients is crucial for diagnosis and treatment – for example, to prevent drug interactions – patients do not always share vital information with their clinician, especially about a medication like sildenafil. It's important for patients to report all medications they are taking, including alternative medicines or over-the-counter medications. It's also important for doctors to use system 2 thinking and to carefully think through a diagnosis and treatment to make sure they are not missing anything or forgetting to ask an important question. That means looking it up.

Hudson turned out to be fine. A cardiologist at the hospital saw him, and the next day, he was sent home. "I told Hudson that the next time he comes to the emergency with chest pain, he should tell us that he was taking Viagra. I guess he may have been a bit too shy to say that he had taken this medication, but it is quite important; it can be life-threatening," Geneviève said.

Chapter 9

The Hidden Problem of Health Literacy

A picture says a thousand words. However, when it comes to health issues, computer screens say much more, whether they have pictures or not.

Julian, a 25-year-old family medicine resident, told Pierre about an experience he had treating a 50-year-old man who had come in complaining about a sore foot. The first thing Julian had to do was decide if an X-ray was necessary. He pulled out his tablet and searched the site Essential Evidence Plus for a clinical decision rule. After he entered the results of his clinical examination, the rule's recommendation was clear: the patient did not require an X-ray. The ankle was probably sprained.

Julian thought it was a pretty black-and-white situation. Unfortunately, the patient didn't. As Julian reported, the patient asked, "Are you sure? I think I need an X-ray." Julian suspected the patient doubted him because he was a resident. "I could have asked my supervisor to speak with him, to reiterate what I had said," Julian said. Instead, he held his hand-held computer up and showed the patient the information he had found. "Just showing him calmed him down," Julian said.

Contrary to what many doctors believe, seeing a doctor use a computer during a medical examination can often make a patient more confident about the doctor's diagnosis and recommended treatment when the information is trustworthy and shared.

Sheila, an experienced 58-year-old family physician who taught residents as part of her medical practice, told Pierre about a house call she made to an elderly woman suffering from lower back pain with sciatic neuralgia (pain in the leg and foot). "The woman was taking both a narcotic painkiller and a muscle relaxant. When I got there, her speech was slurred," Sheila said. "I had a feeling she was taking too much medication."

Sheila knew she had to check the dosages to confirm her suspicion. "In situations like this I always have the choice of information on paper versus computer. On the whole, computers are more convincing." Sheila pulled out her mobile phone and, right in front of her patient, searched Lexi-Drugs (a drug database) for the recommended dosages. She then recommended the patient stop taking the muscle relaxant pills and reduce the dose of her narcotic painkiller. "When I look things up in the paper-printed book, patients look at me like I don't know what I'm doing. But when I use the smart phone, they look at me like, 'Oh! She is up to date.'"

There is nothing really unusual about situations like the ones Sheila and Julian faced. Doctors grapple almost every day with the challenge of how to convince patients what they are recommending is the best solution. Doctors know it's important for patients to understand as much as possible about their diagnosis and treatment, because the more patients understand, the more likely they are to take their medication as instructed and, ultimately, get better.

But explaining medical information to patients and family caregivers is not as simple as it sounds. It boils down to what the medical world refers to as health literacy.

Low literacy is a major concern everywhere, including Canada. Results of a 2011–12 survey of a representative sample of 25,267 Canadians aged 16 to 65 years showed that 49% had a low literacy level: they had difficulty finding, understanding, and using information presented in a dense or lengthy text; navigating complex digital texts; interpreting and evaluating information (constructing meaning); and disregarding irrelevant or inappropriate content when there is competing information (including when the correct content is more prominent).[1] The numbers are very similar in the United States.[1] Furthermore, anybody can face a transitory low literacy level when they are in a stressful situation. The interdependence between information and emotion is well established in the information literature.[2] Literacy is usually rated on a scale of 1 to 5, on the basis of how well participants are able to understand and act on information they are given. For example, about one in 10 Canadians (8.8%) score at literacy level 1 according to the Canadian Council on Learning.[3] Adults at literacy level 1 experience difficulties with very simple text and math (performing below the average level of adults who dropped out of high school and never earned a diploma or its equivalent). At this level, for example, a parent may be unable to determine from a package label the correct dose of a drug to give their child.

Health literacy is quite a different matter. The Canadian Expert Panel on Health Literacy defines it as "the ability to access, understand, evaluate and communicate information as a way to promote, maintain, and improve health in a variety of settings across the life course."[4] Health literacy is a key determinant of health, and it is mobilized for a wide range of daily tasks, such as making healthy lifestyle choices, finding and understanding health and safety information, and locating appropriate health services. Health literacy, computer literacy, and information literacy (literacies) are interdependent. Culture is central to health literacy, and one's literacy level depends on one's ability to understand systems of symbols from the local dominant culture and language. In addition, health literacy level is *situational* and *contextual* given that a social network can compensate for an individual's low literacy level, while stressful circumstances can "decrease" an individual's health literacy level.

One Canadian expert, Linda Shohet, PhD, executive director of the Centre for Literacy in Montreal, became interested in health literacy after realizing that at times she herself didn't seem to have sufficient health literacy skills to navigate the health system. The problem, she says, is that most health information, the way it's normally delivered, is only useful for patients whose literacy skills are at level 4 or 5. "Health is a specific problem, with specific challenges. There's a tremendous mismatch between people's abilities and the difficulty of the material."

The number of people with low skills in health literacy is much higher than the number of people with low skills in regular literacy. According to a study by the Canadian Council on Learning, some 60% of Canadian adults have a low level of health literacy, meaning they have difficulty "acquiring, understanding, and applying health information on their own."[5] For Canadians over 65 years of age, this number climbs to 80%.

In other words, most Canadians cannot actually make sense of complex health information and need help interpreting it. According to a program led by the Organisation for Economic Co-operation and Development (OECD) called the International Adult Literacy and Life Skills (IALS) survey, Canada scored roughly in the middle among industrialized countries in terms of health literacy. The IALS survey looked at how people acted in 190 different health situations.

Many studies on health literacy have concluded that a big problem is simply the way medical information is conveyed, both by doctors and in written materials supplied, say, by pharmaceutical companies. Health consumers with lower levels of health literacy are easily discouraged by information they find difficult to understand.[6] One study on pharmaceutical information concluded that the high reading level and length of drug information leaflets actually discouraged consumers from purchasing medications.[7]

"And that doesn't even take into account the role of emotions," explains Linda Shohet. "When people are trying to understand health information, they are usually under a great deal of stress. Even the most highly literate people can't process information under those circumstances."

Dr Shohet decided to carry out her own study to see how stress affects patients' and families' ability to understand medical information. She put up some very clear and simple information in hospital waiting rooms and then carried out interviews with patients to see what they thought about it. "We assumed the information would be most useful for people with low health literacy, because it was so simple. As it turned out, only the most highly health-literate people read it. They told us they appreciated getting information that was easy to grasp because in a hospital waiting room they were overwhelmed and couldn't deal with anything complex."

Doctors know, at least in theory, how important good communication skills are in helping people get, or stay, healthy. They are taught, for example, how to break bad news. At the end of their studies, family physicians are expected to be able to establish and maintain effective communication in the face of patients' disabilities, cultural differences, and age differences. But the training they actually get is limited and varies widely from one medical school to another.

According to Dr Shohet, time constraints are not the only problem doctors have to contend with and they may not even be the biggest problem. "Health care providers and patients just have very different ideas about what needs to be known. Health care providers think patients want to know *everything*. But patients can't take everything in. They want to know what risks they are facing," she says.

In 2007, the American Medical Association published "six simple methods for improving communication," in the hopes of helping doctors learn to better explain information to their patients.[8] Among the recommendations, doctors were told to "slow down," to use "non-medical language," to ask patients to repeat what they'd been told (to make sure they understood), to limit the amount of information they were giving (not "tell it all"), and "to show or draw pictures." (We will discuss the sixth one later in this chapter.) International consensus is to assume that all patients have a low level of health literacy because of educational and/or socio-cultural and/or emotional reasons.

Using electronic knowledge resources can enable doctors to do these things. "The Internet can provide clear, visual information, but it can also help by providing video and audio material such as simple podcasts. People can watch or hear something over and over, as many times as they need to in order to understand," Dr Shohet confirmed.

Roland, for one, frequently turns to Google images to help patients understand diagnoses and treatment. In one dramatic case, a young man who had recently emigrated from Morocco walked into his clinic complaining of abdominal pain. During the consultation, Roland asked the man about what was going on in his life. The man said he had been under a lot of stress at work lately. Roland suspected the man was suffering from stress-related symptoms, but the patient wasn't convinced. He insisted Roland do an ultrasound.

Roland was glad he heeded his patient's instincts, even though the results of the ultrasound turned out to be devastating. The man had a rare problem called polycystic kidney disease, an inherited disorder that causes clusters of cysts in the kidney. The disease could cause high blood pressure and eventual kidney failure. The only cure would be a kidney transplant.

When the patient returned for a follow-up appointment, Roland knew how hard it would be to explain the condition. Indeed, the man was too emotionally overwhelmed to absorb the information. Roland decided to try to help him with a picture. He did a search on his computer and pulled up an image of a diseased kidney from Google images (comparing a normal kidney with a polycystic kidney).[9] The man wasn't angry or shocked; he was stunned. As he gazed at the image, Roland explained what he really needed to understand: he had to see a nephrologist (a doctor who specializes in treating the kidneys).

While doctors can use their instant access to online images to help their patients understand information, the Internet offers another advantage to heath care professionals and patients. Health care professionals can also use it to organize complex information so their patients can better grasp it.

John, a 55-year-old community pharmacist working in a family health clinic, took advantage of this one day when he was filling out a prescription for Isabella, a woman who had just been diagnosed with rheumatoid arthritis. Isabella's doctor had decided to start treatment with methotrexate. Methotrexate was originally developed to treat cancer, but it was later found to be effective in treating rheumatoid arthritis.

John knew the drug well. Among other things, methotrexate was known to have serious side effects, including bone marrow suppression, which reduces the production of cells that provide immunity and normal blood clotting. As a result, John was hesitant about simply handing Isabella the medication; Isabella had to understand how to handle it all first. John explained to Isabella that methotrexate had to be dosed very carefully. She would have to do frequent tests to check her white blood cells and liver enzymes. If Isabella took this medication, she would have to do blood work every two weeks. "We had to make a monitoring plan for her, so she would know when to do her blood work and know when she might see some side effects," John said.

John had the feeling Isabella might not be ready to take all this information in on the spot. Instead, he gave her some handouts she could take home and read as many times as she needed, and then she could take the time she needed to think it over. "I went to the ecps [the electronic version of the *Compendium of Pharmaceuticals and Specialties*, a comprehensive list of drug monographs]. And then I clicked on the Wyeth Canada one [the monograph provided by the Wyeth pharmaceutical company about their product, as other companies also produce methotrexate]. I printed the handout document for patients and gave it to her."

Isabella took the information home, mulled it over, and decided to start methotrexate after all. "I was confident it was an informed decision and that Isabella would be ready to handle the complex treatment," John told us.

Organizing information is a big part of managing chronic conditions. It will become all the more important as the population ages, and more people develop the chronic conditions associated with aging. Osteoarthritis, for instance, is recognized as one of the most important health problems in the developed world, and it is becoming more common because of the increasing rate of obesity (responsible for the rising incidence of knee osteoarthritis at younger ages) and our longer lifespans. According to the 2010 Canadian Community Health Survey, arthritis and other rheumatic conditions affected nearly 4.5 million Canadians aged 15 years and older (approximately 13% of the entire population). By the year 2025, it is estimated that close to 8 million Canadians will have osteoarthritis. Patients with osteoarthritis usually have to take painkillers and anti-inflammatory drugs; their care can be complicated because they are often taking other drugs, for other diseases, at the same time.

Patients with high blood pressure and diabetes, for example, typically have to manage taking about five medications on a daily basis. There is a lot of information about their medications as well as about the interventions for these conditions that they may eventually need. Many patients with high blood pressure and diabetes who are also obese will eventually develop sleep apnea, osteoarthritis, and chronic pain. Thus, they will have to learn about continuous positive airway pressure as well as treatments for arthritis. The former is the use of positive pressure to maintain an open airway in a spontaneously breathing patient, and it is the most effective treatment for obstructive sleep apnea.

Another obstacle doctors face when they are trying to communicate information to patients is shame. As Linda Shohet puts it, "People don't always ask when they don't understand something. They feel stupid. And they realize their doctor is rushed." In fact, the final recommendation of the American Medical Association's "six simple methods for improving communication" is to create a "shame free environment."

Providing information to patients and family caregivers is relatively easy; the hard part is making sure they understand it. This gets to the heart of the health literacy challenge. Roland often wishes he could evaluate his patients' health literacy skills one by one, but few doctors would have time to conduct such an evaluation.

Still, signs that a patient suffers from very low health literacy can be obvious. Roland recalls a recent immigrant from Jamaica who had to fill out a health insurance form about her diabetes. When Roland asked when she would complete this form, she replied, "My daughter is going to help me." Roland had heard those words before and knew that they were a coping strategy for patients who are illiterate. Patients never say, "I can't do this." It's embarrassing for them. They say, "I'll get help doing this."

But it's not always easy for doctors to tell if a patient has understood information or not. In 28 years of practice, Roland has rarely heard a patient say, "I don't understand." Sometimes Roland suspects they don't, and sometimes he asks. Invariably, patients say "yes" or brush it off. Sometimes Roland asks them to repeat the information he gave them. Very often, they can't.

Electronic knowledge resources can also help overcome the shame barrier. Roland often refers his patients to educational websites, where they can take their time to read and improve their understanding.

Of course, as we saw previously, the Internet can create the opposite problem: patients understand the information so well that they start questioning their doctors' judgment. But Internet information itself can help in this situation too.

James, a 64-year-old writer originally from New York but living in a small town in Northern Ontario, arrived at a health care clinic complaining about lower abdominal pain and frequent loose stools. James saw Jennifer, a middle-aged family physician who worked part-time in the clinic and part-time in the local community hospital. Like James, Jennifer was a fan of outdoor activities, and she often spent weekends at her cottage. She was pretty sure she knew what James was suffering from. She did a stool culture and ordered tests for ova and parasites.

Jennifer received the results a week later. As she suspected, James had giardiasis, otherwise known as beaver fever. Giardiasis is a common intestinal infection caused by a microscopic parasite called *Giardia*. The infection is typically caught in situations where sanitation is poor or where the water is unsafe to drink, like backcountry lakes. The symptoms – abdominal pain, nausea, and diarrhea – mean giardiasis can be confused with other infections such as gastroenteritis, otherwise known as stomach flu.

Like stomach flu, giardiasis can just disappear without being treated. However, if the symptoms last for more than a few days, like in James' case, it's best to treat it. The problem is that treatment for giardiasis has been a controversial topic for the last 30 years. Some studies have concluded that a one-day treatment is usually enough, whereas others recommend a three- to seven-day treatment because this length of treatment is almost 100% effective.

After looking on Essential Evidence Plus, Jennifer decided to prescribe a five-day treatment with metronidazole. James looked it up and refused to accept her recommendation. "James was an intellectual. He wanted lots of information, and I had to answer all his questions first," Jennifer said.

The solution? "In this case, I decided to give him all the literature and let him mull it over himself." That was possible, of course, because all she had to do was to quickly print out what she had found online. In the end, James accepted her recommendation. "I let James know that I'm a very careful clinician, conscientious, and I looked stuff up for him. In the end, that's what made him accept my recommendation."

By making information clear and making it possible to deliver information to patients on the spot, electronic knowledge resources help get patients on board for treatments, or even back on board after they have given up a treatment. Jack, a young family physician working on the West Coast, saw how this worked with Justin, a 45-year-old patient who came into an evening walk-in clinic where he worked.

Justin had been in a motor vehicle accident about six months earlier. He came into Jack's clinic complaining of chronic neck pain. An earlier physician had prescribed an exercise plan for Justin. Justin had tried it for a while but stopped because it didn't seem to be working. If anything, his neck hurt more than when he started the plan.

Jack knew this was a common problem for people suffering from chronic neck pain. "Patients with neck pain often complain of increased pain and don't want to do their exercises," he said. "Traditionally doctors say, 'Well if the exercise hurts, don't do it.'" But Jack decided to look into it and searched Essential Evidence Plus for neck pain. "The site gave me specific instructions to recommend patients do the exercises *despite* the pain."

Jack knew he would have to have compelling information to convince Justin to go back to his painful exercise regime. So he pulled up a synopsis of a study of 180 female office workers with chronic, nonspecific neck pain. The workers were randomly assigned either to one of two training groups or to a control group, with 60 women in each group. The endurance-training group performed dynamic neck exercises, which included lifting the head up from the supine and prone positions. The strength-training group performed high-intensity isometric neck strengthening (muscle contractions without movement) and stabilization exercises with an elastic band.

Both training groups performed dynamic exercises for the shoulders and upper extremities with dumbbells. All groups were advised to do aerobic and stretching exercises three times a week. At the 12-month follow-up visit, both neck pain and disability had decreased in both training groups compared with the control group.[10]

"I pulled this information up and showed Justin the research on exercise programs. I told him it was very important to keep doing the exercise even if it hurt. Justin was more willing to keep doing the active exercise program after that."

When we think about prescriptions we usually think of medications. But more and more, doctors are helping patients by "prescribing" information, recommending websites that provide texts or online videos that patients can consult.

Prescribing information is still a relatively new trend. Over the last decade, a number of studies have tried to determine how effective it is. The results are encouraging. In 2005, 92 self-selected physicians and 907 non-randomly selected patients from 30 different American states participated in a survey on patients' attitudes about information prescriptions and patient-physician communication.[11] Almost all (93%) of the patients reported that the information they found had helped them make better health decisions. A majority (70%) reported that the information they found had improved their understanding of an illness or a health condition. Almost half (45%) reported that the information they found might have influenced their future health decisions.

Far from creating an impression that doctors are sending patients away to do their own work, information prescriptions seem to increase patients' trust in doctors. In the same survey, 84% of patients stated that they were more inclined to trust the information on the Internet resource MedlinePlus because their physician prescribed it to them. Similarly, the physicians who participated in the survey said patients who received an information prescription were likely to feel more comfortable discussing their conditions with them. One physician, Minnesota-based Joan Goering, reported, "My patients were happy to have an address for valid medical information. They felt more comfortable discussing their diagnosis after reading the material on MedlinePlus and seemed to have better questions."

There's no doubt that patients on the whole are more and more likely to look for medical information themselves. We asked Francesca Frati, a medical librarian, about this. Frati works at the library of a teaching hospital in Montreal, where she manages the hospital's Patient & Family Resource Centre. The library and centre provide trustworthy, up-to-date health information for both health professionals and patients. Doctors can refer patients to her, and she will spend the time they need, sometimes up to an hour, she says, finding trustworthy information.

Although most hospitals have medical libraries, surprisingly few patients know about hospital librarians. What motivates people to seek out the help of an information specialist? Two types of patients began advocating for access to information: patients with cancer and patients with AIDS (acquired immune deficiency syndrome). "There were diseases people felt they needed information about, and they weren't getting it," explains Frati. "AIDS, because it was so stigmatized, and cancer, because not too long ago, there was a taboo about it too." Frati also had experience working in a family medicine clinic, where the most common requests for patient information were for topics such as immunization, prenatal care, and nutrition.

Today, more and more patients and their relatives are accessing the Patient & Family Resource Centre's electronic knowledge resources. "Most people use our resources without ever speaking to us," Frati says. "The right integrated approach can be more effective; people are becoming more aware of that. We provide access to research that shows whether an alternative treatment is effective or potentially dangerous to use."

Going through the Patient & Family Resource Centre for information helps solve one big problem health consumers face: finding reliable sources. "There's a lot of bad stuff out there. There's a lot of biased information that looks neutral but is really funded by a pharmaceutical company or written by an activist for a particular cause. If a person doesn't know how to navigate it, they could end up on a website that says baking soda will cure your cancer." To help patients find trustworthy information on their own, Frati tells them about the Health on the Net Foundation, an organization that grants accreditation to health sites.

Over the last decade Frati has seen both doctors' and patients' attitudes about information change. "When I started, doctors still felt a bit threatened by Google, but it's less so now. There are still people who 'don't want to know' and let doctors make the decision, but it's becoming less common." More and more, people who want to take control of their health are going online, she says. "I have some people so far advanced in their knowledge of their disease that they are interested in a professional level of information; they want to look at research. Some of them already know everything there is to deal with."

Increasing comfort with looking for online medical information means more and more patients and family caregivers will turn to the Internet, whether to get information on their own or to better understand information a doctor has "prescribed." Relatives and social network members can help patients to overcome their individual health literacy barriers when needed, to look for and understand information, to manage a health problem, and to navigate the health care system.[12]

Chapter 10

The Family Doctor of the Future

Imagine we are in the year 2035. The medical world is literally paperless. The young doctors who work in clinics and hospitals now have never even seen medical records on paper.

For the last 10 years, since about 2025, all medical students have done all their training using electronic knowledge resources. In 2035, doctors turn to their mobile devices in many consultations to use a brief information needs assessment checklist for both clinicians and patients. The checklist reminds them to find current clinical practice guidelines; check for possible harmful drug interactions; check the latest recommended dosages; read the bottom lines of the newest syntheses of original research studies pertinent to their patient; provide their patient and family members with an appropriate, reliable information source; and more.

In short, doctors now have the latest information the scientific world has to offer about health promotion, disease prevention, diagnosis, medical treatment, and health and social care at their fingertips. They can not only use this information themselves but also share it with a multidisciplinary primary care team, their patients, and family caregivers.

And they use it.

In 2035, doctors are no longer worried about what their patients think when they "look it up." Patients are used to watching their doctors scrolling screens for trustworthy information. In fact, they expect them to do this. Patients who receive an information prescription now sign a form saying they did so and acknowledging that they were asked to use at least one specific patient information source by themselves or with the help of someone else.

Let's take a look at what the consultation of the future will look like. Our patient is Karim, a 52-year-old man who lives in the mid-sized city of Hamilton, Ontario. Karim moved to Canada from Egypt as a teenager, went to school and university in Canada, and became a high school gym teacher. He is married with four teenaged children.

Except for being a few pounds overweight, Karim is in good health. A few years ago, his doctor told him he had hypercholesterolemia (high blood cholesterol) so he cut down on the fat in his diet. He still likes good food and wine, but he compensates for it by watching his diet and staying active. Karim is an avid long-distance runner.

Like most men his age, Karim avoids going to doctors' offices or hospitals as much as possible. The last time Karim saw a doctor was five years ago, to have a hernia repaired. For the last few months, Karim's wife, Norma, has been urging him to make an appointment at their local clinic, not because Karim has particular symptoms but rather because of something she discovered. While she was waiting at the doctor's office for an appointment, Norma watched a documentary about hepatitis C on the clinic's TV network. The show explained that people from the Middle East were at higher risk of having contracted hepatitis C as children than people born and raised in North America. Norma suddenly got worried that Karim might have been one of those children.

Hepatitis C is a disease caused by a virus that affects the liver. It is transmitted when a tiny amount of blood from an infected person gets into the bloodstream of an uninfected person.

Some people who get the virus clear it from their bodies on their own, while others go on to develop serious liver disease from chronic infection. Chronic hepatitis C infection can cause death from cirrhosis (permanent liver scarring) or liver cancer.

Symptoms of chronic hepatitis C include fatigue, nausea, muscle pain, weight loss, and eventually jaundice and pain if cancer develops. The problem is that in its early stages, the disease doesn't have any symptoms. That's the main reason that while an estimated 1% of all Canadians have hepatitis C, one in five of these people don't know it. By the time symptoms appear, it's often too late. Hepatitis can silently affect the liver for 30 years or so before cirrhosis or cancer develops.

Normally, the chances of Karim having caught hepatitis C would have been quite slim. The disease is most frequently transmitted through used needles, and in North America it is most commonly seen among intravenous drug users. But as the documentary explained, immigrants from certain countries, including Egypt, have a higher than normal risk of having contracted it before they emigrated to Canada, either from their mother at childbirth or after they received an injection with a contaminated needle.

Egypt, Norma learned, is one of the countries where children are at higher risk. Norma thought it was a good idea for Karim to find out if he had the virus now rather than later. All he needed to do was have a blood test. After months of gentle reminders, she started to lose patience, and the reminders got less gentle. Eventually, Karim decides to take the afternoon off work and head to the clinic to discuss it with a doctor.

When he goes to his local family health clinic, Karim is seen by Olivia, a 30-year-old doctor who had been practising family medicine for three years. Remember, we are in 2035. Olivia did all her medical training with a mobile device in her hand. As in all other clinics at this time, there are no paper records where she works. The first thing Olivia does when she meets Karim is to open his electronic medical record (EMR) on her smart phone. In 2035, everyone has an EMR, and they contain a lot more than patient information. As part of each patient's EMR, doctors receive updates and alerts about new treatment recommendations, new diagnostic tests, drug interactions, dosage updates, and more.

When Olivia opens Karim's EMR, an alert about hepatitis C pops up. This might seem like science fiction, but it's not. Months before seeing Karim, Olivia had received a POEM with information about the recommendation of the US Preventive Services Task Force (USPSTF) concerning hepatitis C screening for people from other countries. Olivia sees a lot of patients from the Middle East and Africa, so she had set a personalized alert on her mobile device to remind her of this POEM about specific diseases or conditions that might affect this clientele in particular.

Karim is part of that group of patients, so when Olivia opens Karim's EMR, the first thing she sees is the alert about hepatitis C. She then taps a panel on the right side of the screen where she files her "favourites." She scrolls down her list to hepatitis, where there is a link to the USPSTF recommendations. She quickly reads a synopsis of the recommendations and shows Karim her screen, which displays a simple, brief, evidence-based patient-information fact-sheet (including a podcast in several languages). Then she takes a couple of minutes to discuss with Karim the possibility of having a blood test and explains the steps he has to take if the test result is positive.

In other words, in 2035, thanks to Internet technology, a family physician like Olivia will be able to automatically link her continuing medical education resources, which keep her aware of up-to-date research, to individual patients' EMRs where they are relevant. She will only need to spend about a minute getting up to date on the latest clinical guidelines for her patients. She can use all of this information to make informed or shared decisions with her patients about whether to go ahead with tests or treatments or not.

In 2003, doctors at Partners HealthCare in Boston and at the Harvard Medical School wrote "Ten Commandments for Effective Clinical Decision Support: Making the Practice of Evidence-based Medicine a Reality," in which they evaluated how much progress had – and hadn't – been made in getting doctors to use electronic knowledge resources.[1] They also explored the obstacles doctors were still facing.

The authors had high expectations about how technology could change the way they and other clinicians would be able to carry out their work. They wrote the article partly because those expectations hadn't yet been met.

In 2003, they concluded, there were lots of things preventing doctors from using the Internet. One of the biggest problems was time. There was a lot of information available electronically, but it was still hard to locate, and clinicians didn't have enough time to spend searching the Internet during patient consultations.

Even a decade later, in 2015, time was still one of the main obstacles preventing doctors from looking things up. As we wrote in a paper that year, "The environment of primary care medicine severely limits time for searches for clinical information. At the point of care, and given the time required for searches, using electronic knowledge resources during the consultation is perceived to be a complex task."[2] In short, doctors still thought it was complicated to look things up, so they often didn't bother.

We are confident that by 2035, the speed issue will have been solved. Informing patients and family caregivers will become a requirement and a collective responsibility of the primary health care team. Doctors will have all the tools they need to do this quickly and effectively. Doctors like Olivia won't even need to type in passwords to get access to information by this time – access to databases will be biometric, such as via fingerprints – and systems will work rapidly. In her patients' EMRs Olivia will have a panel with information on topics she has chosen to follow, so she can retrieve information quickly at the point of care when she needs it instead of having to start a search from scratch. She will also be able to ask for help from the other members of the primary health care team where she is working.

Olivia's "favourites" list will, of course, start to get pretty long after a while, but the EMRs will have solutions to that problem, too. EMRs will have built-in search engines specifically to retrieve information from clinicians' lists of favourite content. The recommendations will be organized by date, so she can see what, if anything, is new in the past year. If a study is obsolete, the EMR will "tell" her. That means Olivia will be able to find what she needs quickly and efficiently, and this will give her the time she needs to share whatever pertinent information she finds for each patient, not only with her patients but also with her team, improving interprofessional communication and coordination.

Another problem the authors of the "Ten Commandments" article found back in 2003 was that information had to be packaged much more concisely than it was at the time, or doctors wouldn't make use of it. "You need to fit a guideline on a single screen for people to use it," the authors wrote.

We believe that problem will be solved by 2035 as well. Primary care clinicians will no longer have to plow through lengthy guideline statements. Instead, they'll receive, and easily be able to locate subsequently, brief highlights with updated clinical recommendations. There will be a systematic mechanism to identity all new guidelines and extract all the new recommendations.

The authors of the "Ten Commandments" article identified yet another problem in 2003. They called it the problem of "fitting consultation of electronic knowledge resources into doctors' workflow." The problem was that if a doctor came across a recommendation to do something, she might read it. But she might only *need* it in a week, or a month, or more. So how could doctors possibly remember to apply the information to their patients when they needed to?

In 2035, doctors, nurse practitioners, and pharmacists won't use mobile devices just to "look it up." They'll also use their devices to "take it in." Updated information will flow into clinicians' laptops and onto their mobile devices every day. Clinicians will start the day with a quick glance at their phone to see what's there. They won't be worried about information overload because the information will be automatically directed where it belongs, into their own "favourites" files and directly into patients' EMRs, which they will access on their hand-held device. In other words, clinicians will have a personalized, accessible online information "library" at their fingertips.

Some might wonder whether this new automated world of information will create a medical world that is dominated by artificial intelligence, where doctors – if we even need them anymore – will just repeat what the machines say. On the contrary, as more information becomes readily available, doctors, nurses, pharmacists, and allied health professionals will become more important as the interpreters of that information in accordance with the specific clinical and social history, values, and preferences of the patient and her or his family. No matter how sophisticated and well programmed they are, machines cannot offer much contextual judgment without analyzing a large amount of data. Medicine is about people in specific situations. Computers are about patterns. Unsupervised machine learning (deep learning) dramatically increases the discovery and recognition of patterns, but if we imagined robots diagnosing people, they would only be able to recognize patterns.[3] As Will Knight (senior editor for artificial intelligence and robotics at the journal *MIT Technology Review*) put it, "it is hard to envision how we will collaborate with [increasingly sophisticated and complex artificial intelligence systems] without language, i.e., without being able to ask them 'Why?' More than this, the ability to communicate effortlessly with computers would make them infinitely more useful."[4]

Clinicians don't necessarily follow patterns when they make a diagnosis; when they communicate with patients and relatives to make sense of their patients' clinical situation; and when they interpret diverse forms of evidence from multiple sources (as we mentioned in the introduction) in the context of specific situations, using intuition and mindlines. Each clinical case has idiosyncratic elements that have to be interpreted with the patient and with other members of their family. A clinician uses her experience and knowledge of the person in front of her; for instance, she uses her understanding of how her patient may differ from the people included in randomized controlled trials (the very elderly, for example, are rarely chosen to participate in drug trials). In other words, medical knowledge, no matter how accessible and trustworthy, is only useful as part of a conversation between patients and clinicians. A machine can't register the unique situation of any human being and the tacit exchange of non-codified knowledge between clinicians and patients. It can only "talk" to other machines using codified knowledge (information). To start a machine learning program would require that a massive number of patient-clinician interactions be recorded; even then, computers scientists would need clinicians to interpret the patterns the machine observed. Herbert Simon, a famous pioneer of artificial intelligence and scholar in behavioural sciences and management (a "father" of bounded rationality and organizational learning), described this paradox in the 1950s: for managing complex situations, it is more efficient to invest in experts than in programmers.[5] Typically, many clinical encounters are complex, and many patients have complex primary care (health and social) needs, which will be more efficiently managed by clinicians rather than machines.

But this question remains: Will clinicians be able to adapt to the radical shift that is underway, in which a constant flow of new medical information will be part of their day-to-day practice? We think this challenge can be met with a system we have been working on, in partnership with the College of Family Physicians of Canada and the Canadian Medical Association. It's called the Information Assessment Method, or IAM. The IAM is a questionnaire that clinicians fill out to evaluate information updates they receive, like POEMS.

Let's go back to our story about Olivia and Karim to see how this might work. Say Olivia has been using the IAM since she started practising medicine. She has been filling out the IAM questionnaire in part because this process helps her to meet the requirement for continuing medical education in her medical specialty.

But filling out the questionnaire does more than fulfill her training requirements. Using the IAM questionnaire actually helps Olivia gather and organize information on a day-to-day basis. By using it, Olivia can tag any recommendations she thinks will be useful for her practice. She has an app that automatically transfers recommendations and other information she tags to the EMRs of patients for whom the information will be relevant. She has established criteria to determine which information will be useful for which patients, on the basis of things like the patient's age, sex, chronic conditions they have, and their background (such as breast cancer in the family). In Karim's case one of the criteria is his birthplace, which puts him at higher risk for hepatitis C.

For clinicians like Olivia, keeping up to date about new information will be part of their daily routine. Olivia will get up in the morning, have a coffee, and open her mobile device to check her alerts, the same way people now check their email at the start of the day. Each alert will be linked to a clinical pathway with information on diagnoses and treatments for specific conditions.

We believe such a system will help clinicians tackle another challenge the authors of the "Ten Commandments" article identified in 2003: finding a balance between under-alerting and over-alerting. A decade after the "Ten Commandments" authors identified this problem, clinicians were still overwhelmed by the number of emails coming in with new information and recommendations. Clinicians were receiving thousands of clinical recommendations every year, and since they didn't know how to wade through them, let alone keep track of the ones they might need, they tended to ignore them.

How will the IAM questionnaire solve the problem of being overwhelmed by too much information? It will allow clinicians to set automatic alerts to identify, then organize, information about specific subjects relevant to them and their practice. Clinicians can then store that information for the future in a way that they will easily be able to find it when they need it. Clinicians using the system have already told us they find it a more efficient way of staying up to date and that it helps them apply recommendations that they themselves have identified as being beneficial for their patients.

Clinics in the future will also be able to use technology to make clinician-patient communication fast and efficient. When Olivia views Karim's test results, all she will have to do is click a button on her hand-held device to automatically send an email to Karim to let him know that the results were negative.

Like most doctors of her time, Olivia will know it's more important than ever to be able to find information quickly. By all estimates, primary health care demands will have increased further by 2035. As the population ages, more people will be living with chronic diseases. More tests and more treatments will be available. There will also be more information available about diseases, and more interdisciplinary team members will be available to give information and feedback to patients and family caregivers.

In short, clinicians will have to be able to handle information quickly and effectively. Their ability to remain up to date and find the information quickly when they need it will help them to deliver better care, prevent mistakes, and save more lives.

The year 2035 sounds to us like an ideal world. We're confident it will only take another 20 years for this to become a reality.

Notes

Introduction

1 Hersh, *Information-Retrieval*; and Pluye et al., "Information-Retrieval Technology."
2 Pluye et al., "Situational Relevance"; Pluye et al., "Using Electronic Knowledge Resources (Part 1)"; Pluye et al., "Number Needed to Benefit"; Pluye et al., "Four Levels of Outcomes"; and Pluye et al., "Comprehensive and Systematic Information Assessment Method."
3 Bindiganavile Sridhar, Pluye, and Grad, "Information Assessment"; and Badran, "Information Assessment Method."
4 Grad et al., "Value of Therapeutic Information."
5 Grad et al., "Big Data."
6 Saracevic and Kantor, "Value of Library and Information Services."
7 Pluye et al., "Four Levels of Outcomes."
8 Pluye and Hong, "Combining the Power of Stories and the Power of Numbers."
9 Canadian Institutes of Health Research, "Knowledge Translation."
10 Pluye et al., "Number Needed to Benefit"; Pluye et al., "Four Levels of Outcomes"; and Pluye et al., "Using Electronic Knowledge Resources (Part 2)."

11 Pluye et al., "Number Needed to Benefit."

12 Pluye et al., "Number Needed to Benefit"; Pluye et al., "Four Levels of Outcomes"; and Pluye et al., "Using Electronic Knowledge Resources (Part 2)."

13 Sackett et al., "Evidence-Based Medicine."

14 Heath, "How Medicine Has Exploited Rationality."

15 Feinstein, "Clinical Judgment."

16 Greenhalgh et al., "Open Letter."

17 Greenhalgh, Howick, and Maskrey, "Evidence Based Medicine."

18 Luhmann, *Social Systems*; and Luhmann, "What Is Communication?"

19 OCEBM Table of Evidence Working Group et al., "Levels of Evidence"; and Brownson, Roux and Swartz, "Rigorous Evidence for Public Health."

Chapter One

1 Kahane, Stutz, and Aliarzadeh, "Be All-Knowing."

2 Ely et al., "Answering Doctors' Questions."

3 Del Fiol, Workman, and Gorman, "Clinical Questions."

4 McGaha et al., "Medical Students' Frequently Asked Questions."

5 Kahane, Stutz, and Aliarzadeh, "Be All-Knowing."

6 Stern, "Measuring Medical Professionalism."

7 Gurteen, "Quotation."

Chapter Two

1 Siegel, Miller, and Jemal, "Cancer Statistics."

2 National Lung Screening Trial Research Team, "Lung-Cancer Mortality."

3 Welch, "Overdiagnosed."

4 Bleyer and Welch, "Screening Mammography."

5 Evans, McAllister, and Sanders, "Coeliac Disease."

6 Fasano, "Coeliac Disease"; and Fasano and Catassi, "Clinical Practice."

7 Légaré and Witteman, "Shared Decision Making."
8 Légaré et al., "Validating a Conceptual Model."
9 Charles, Gafni, and Whelan, "Decision-Making in the Physician-Patient Encounter."
10 Veroff, Marr, and Wennberg, "Support for Shared Decision Making."
11 Donnelly, Shaw, and van den Akker, "Ehealth as a Challenge."

Chapter Three

1 White, "Evidence-Based Medicine."
2 College of Family Physicians of Canada, "Competency Based Curriculum."
3 Malcolm, Wong, and Elwood-Martin, "Patients' Perceptions."
4 Pineault et al., "Solo Practices."
5 Haggerty et al., "Continuity of Care."
6 Agency for Healthcare Research and Quality, "Nurse Practitioners."
7 Roots and MacDonald, "Nurse Practitioners in Collaborative Practice."

Chapter Four

1 Statistics Canada, "Health State Descriptions."
2 Canadian Institute for Health Information, "Drug Use among Seniors."
3 Liu and Christensen, "Inappropriate Prescribing."
4 Comissaire à la santé et au bien-être Québec, "Les Médicaments."
5 Beales et al., "Exploring Professional Culture."
6 Jorgenson et al., "Pharmacists Teaching."
7 Beales et al., "Exploring Professional Culture."

Chapter Five

1 Ahmad, "Adverse Drug Event Monitoring."
2 Health Canada, "Canada Vigilance."
3 Grad et al., "Value of Clinical Information."

4 Ioannidis, "Highly Cited Clinical Research"; and Contopoulos-Ioannidis et al., "Translational Research."
5 de Haen et al., "Efficacy of Duct Tape."
6 Wellbery and McAteer, "Avoiding Practice Pitfalls."
7 Bruggink et al., "Cutaneous Warts."
8 Slawson, Shaughnessy, and Bennett, "Medical Information Master."
9 Slawson and Shaughnessy, "Teaching Evidence-Based Medicine."
10 Slawson, "Teaching Evidence-Based Medicine."
11 Haynes et al., "McMaster Plus."
12 Roger et al., "Heart Disease and Stroke."
13 Radley, Finkelstein, and Stafford, "Off-Label Prescribing."

Chapter Six

1 Landro, "Less Can Be More."
2 Pluye et al., "Using Electronic Knowledge Resources (Part 2)"; Pluye et al., "Number Needed to Benefit"; Pluye et al., "Four Levels of Outcomes"; and Westbrook et al., "Critical Incidents."
3 Hersh et al., "Success in Searching MEDLINE"; Hersh et al., "Successful Answering of Clinical Questions"; Labrecque et al., "Decision Making in Family Medicine"; McKibbon and Fridsma, "Clinician-Selected Electronic Information"; McKibbon et al., "Correct Answers"; Westbrook, Coiera, and Gosling, "Online Information Retrieval Systems"; Rouleau, Gagnon, and Côté, "Information and Communication Technologies"; and Pluye et al., "Information-Retrieval Technology."
4 Tonsaker, Bartlett, and Trpkov, "Health Information."
5 Légaré and Witteman, "Shared Decision Making"; and Légaré et al., "Implementing Shared Decision-Making."

Chapter Seven

1 Statistics Canada, "Canadian Internet Use."
2 Anderson and Perrin, "Americans Who Don't Use the Internet."
3 Tu and Cohen, "Consumers Seeking Health Care Information."
4 Lavoie and Fontaine, "Parentalité au Québec."

5 Chatman, "Impoverished Life-World."
6 White and Horvitz, "Cyberchondria."
7 White and Horvitz, "Experiences with Web Search."
8 Pluye et al., "Online Parenting Information."
9 Pluye et al., "Development and Content Validation."
10 Tonsaker, Bartlett, and Trpkov, "Health Information."
11 Hersh et al., "Success in Searching Medline"; Hersh et al., "Successful Answering of Clinical Questions"; Labrecque et al., "Decision Making in Family Medicine"; McKibbon and Fridsma, "Clinician-Selected Electronic Information"; McKibbon et al., "Correct Answers"; and Westbrook, Coiera, and Gosling, "Online Information Retrieval Systems."

Chapter Eight

1 Gabbay and le May, "Guidelines and Mindlines."
2 Kahneman, *Thinking Fast and Slow.*
3 Berner, "Decision Support Systems"; and Sullivan and MacNaughton, "Evidence in Consultations."
4 Tamblyn et al., "Medical Office."

Chapter Nine

1 Organisation for Economic Co-operation and Development, "Skills Outlook."
2 Nahl and Bilal, *Information and Emotion*; and Nahl, "Social–Biological Information Technology."
3 Canadian Council on Learning, "Health Literacy."
4 McNichol and Rootman, "Literacy and Health Literacy."
5 Canadian Council on Learning, "Health Literacy."
6 Bennett et al., "Contribution of Health Literacy."
7 Winterstein et al., "Consumer Medication Information."
8 Weiss and Schwartzberg, *Health Literacy.*
9 The Google image comparing a normal kidney with a polycystic kidney was produced by the Mayo Foundation for Medical Education and Research. www.google.ca/search?q=polycystic+kidney+

disease&tbm=isch&ved=0ahUKEwjXjceolvzQAhXG6YM
KHavNCAwQ_AUICCgB#imgrc=w47nKxvJkrGs3M%3A
(accessed 27 November 2016).

10 Ylinen et al., "Treatment of Chronic Neck Pain."
11 Siegel et al., "Information Rx."
12 Pluye et al., "Development and Content Validation."

Chapter Ten

1 Bates et al., "Effective Clinical Decision Support."
2 Grad et al., "Do Family Physicians Retrieve Synopses."
3 Goodfellow, Bengio, and Courville, *Deep Learning*.
4 Knight, "AI's Language Problem."
5 Simon, *Sciences of the Artificial*.

Bibliography

Agency for Healthcare Research and Quality. "The Number of Nurse
    Practitioners and Physician Assistants Practicing Primary Care in
    the United States. Primary Care Workforce Facts and Stats No. 2."
    Rockville, MD: Agency for Healthcare Research and Quality, 2012.
    www.ahrq.gov/research/findings/factsheets/primary/pcwork2/
    index.html (accessed 27 November 2016).

Ahmad, S.R. "Adverse Drug Event Monitoring at the Food and Drug
    Administration." *Journal of General Internal Medicine* 18, no. 1
    (2003): 57–60, doi:10.1046/j.1525-1497.2003.20130.x.

Anderson, M., and A. Perrin. "13% of Americans Don't Use the
    Internet: Who Are They?" Washington, DC: Pew Research Center,
    7 September 2016. www.pewresearch.org/fact-tank/2016/09/07/
    some-americans-dont-use-the-internet-who-are-they (accessed 27
    November 2016).

Badran, H. "Content Validation of the Information Assessment
    Method for Delivery of Educational Material: A Mixed Methods
    Study." MSc thesis, McGill University, 2014. http://digitool.Library.
    McGill.CA:80/R/-?func=dbin-jump-full&object_id=127224&silo_
    library=GEN01 (accessed 27 November 2016).

Bates, D.W., G.J. Kuperman, S. Wang, T. Gandhi, A. Kittler, L. Volk, C. Spurr, et al. "Ten Commandments for Effective Clinical Decision Support: Making the Practice of Evidence-Based Medicine a Reality." *Journal of the American Medical Informatics Association* 10, no. 6 (2003): 523–30, doi:10.1197/jamia.M1370.

Beales, J., R. Walji, C. Papoushek, and Z. Austin. "Exploring Professional Culture in the Context of Family Health Team Interprofessional Collaboration." *Health and Interprofessional Practice* 1, no. 1 (2011): eP1004, doi:10.7772/2159-1253.1012.

Bennett, I.M., J. Chen, J.S. Soroui, and S. White. "The Contribution of Health Literacy to Disparities in Self-Rated Health Status and Preventive Health Behaviors in Older Adults." *Annals of Family Medicine* 7, no. 3 (2009): 204–11, doi:10.1370/afm.940.

Berner, E.S. "Clinical Decision Support Systems: State of the Art." AHRQ Publication no. 90069. Rockville, MD: Agency for Healthcare Research and Quality, 2009.

Bindiganavile Sridhar, S., P. Pluye, and R. Grad. "In Pursuit of a Valid Information Assessment Method for Continuing Education: A Mixed Methods Study." *BMC Medical Education* 13 (2013): 137, doi:10.1186/1472-6920-13-137.

Bleyer, A., and H.G. Welch. "Effect of Three Decades of Screening Mammography on Breast-Cancer Incidence." *New England Journal of Medicine* 367, no. 12 (2012): 1998–2005, doi:10.1056/NEJMoa1206809.

Brownson, R.C., A.V.D. Roux, and K. Swartz. "Commentary: Generating Rigorous Evidence for Public Health: The Need for New Thinking to Improve Research and Practice." *Annual Review of Public Health* 35, no. 1 (2014): 1–7, doi:10.1146/annurev-publhealth-112613-011646.

Bruggink, S.C., J.A. Eekhof, P.F. Egberts, S.C. van Blijswijk, W.J. Assendelft, and J. Gus.sekloo. "Natural Course of Cutaneous Warts among Primary Schoolchildren: A Prospective Cohort Study." *Annals of Family Medicine* 11, no. 5 (2013): 437–41, doi:10.1370/afm.1508.

Canadian Council on Learning. "Health Literacy in Canada: A
Healthy Understanding." Ottawa: Canadian Council on Learning,
2008. www.bth.se/hal/halsoteknik.nsf/bilagor/HealthLiteracy
ReportFeb2008E_pdf/$file/HealthLiteracyReportFeb2008E.pdf.

Canadian Institute for Health Information. "Drug Use among Seniors
on Public Drug Programs in Canada, 2002 to 2008." Ottawa: Canadian Institute for Health Information, 2010. https://secure.cihi.ca/
free_products/drug_use_in_seniors_2002-2008_e.pdf (accessed
27 November 2016).

Canadian Institutes of Health Research. "Knowledge Translation."
Ottawa: Canadian Institutes of Health Research. www.cihr-irsc.
gc.ca/e/29418.html (accessed 27 November 2016).

Charles, C., A. Gafni, and T. Whelan. "Decision-Making in the
Physician-Patient Encounter: Revisiting the Shared Treatment
Decision-Making Model." *Social Science and Medicine* 49, no. 5
(1999): 651–61, doi:10.1016/S0277-9536(99)00145-8.

Chatman, E.A. "The Impoverished Life-World of Outsiders." *Journal
of the Association for Information Science and Technology* 47, no. 3
(1996):193–206,doi:10.1002(SICI)1097-4571(199603)47:3<193::AID-
ASI3>3.0.CO;2-T.

College of Family Physicians of Canada. "Triple C Competency Based
Curriculum [Canmeds-Fm: A Framework of Competencies in
Family Medicine]." Mississauga, ON: College of Family Physicians
of Canada. www.cfpc.ca/Triple_C (accessed 27 November 2016).

Comissaire à la santé et au bien-être Québec. "Les Médicaments D'or-
donnance: Etat de la Situation au Québec (Deuxième Version)."
Québec: Comissaire à la santé et au bien-être Québec. www.csbe.
gouv.qc.ca/fileadmin/www/2014/Medicaments/CSBE_Medica
ments_EtatSituation_2e.pdf (accessed 27 November 2016).

Contopoulos-Ioannidis, D.G., G.A. Alexiou, T.C. Gouvias, and J.P.A.
Ioannidis. "Life Cycle of Translational Research for Medical Interventions." *Science* 321 (2008): 1298–9, doi:10.1126/science.1160622.

de Haen, M., M.G. Spigt, C.J. van Uden, P. van Neer, F.J. Feron, and A.
Knottnerus. "Efficacy of Duct Tape vs Placebo in the Treatment of

Verruca vulgaris (Warts) in Primary School Children." *Archives of Pediatrics and Adolescent Medicine* 160 (2006): 1121–5, doi:10.1001/archpedi.160.11.1121.

Del Fiol, G., T.E. Workman, and P.N. Gorman. "Clinical Questions Raised by Clinicians at the Point of Care: A Systematic Review." *Journal of the American Medical Association Internal Medicine* 174, no. 5 (2014): 710–8, doi:10.1001/jamainternmed.2014.368.

Donnelly, L.S., R.L. Shaw, and O.B. van den Akker. "Ehealth as a Challenge to 'Expert' Power: A Focus Group Study of Internet Use for Health Information and Management." *Journal of the Royal Society of Medicine* 101, no. 10 (2008): 501–6, doi:10.1258/jrsm.2008.080156.

Ely, J.W., J.A. Osheroff, M.H. Ebell, M.L. Chambliss, D.C. Vinson, J.J. Stevermer, and E.A. Pifer. "Obstacles to Answering Doctors' Questions about Patient Care with Evidence: Qualitative Study." *British Medical Journal* 324 (2002), doi:10.1136/bmj.324.7339.710.

Evans, K.E., R. McAllister, and D.S. Sanders. "Should We Screen for Coeliac Disease? No." *British Medical Journal* 339 (2009), doi:10.1136/bmj.b3674.

Fasano, A. "Should We Screen for Coeliac Disease? Yes." *British Medical Journal* 339 (2009), doi:10.1136/bmj.b3592.

Fasano, A., and C. Catassi. "Clinical Practice. Celiac Disease." *New England Journal of Medicine* 367, no. 25 (2012): 2419–26, doi:10.1056/NEJMcp1113994.

Feinstein, A.R. "Clinical Judgment Revisited: The Distraction of Quantitative Models." *Annals of Internal Medicine* 120, no. 9 (1994): 799–805, doi:10.7326/0003-4819-120-9-199405010-00012.

Gabbay, J., and A. le May. "Evidence-Based Guidelines or Collectively Constructed 'Mindlines?' Ethnographic Study of Knowledge Management in Primary Care." *British Medical Journal* 329, no. 7473 (2004): e1013, doi:10.1136/bmj.329.7473.1013.

Goodfellow, I., Y. Bengio, and A. Courville. *Deep Learning*. Cambridge, MA: MIT Press, 2016.

Grad, R.M., P. Pluye, V. Granikov, J. Johnson-Lafleur, M. Shulha, S. Bindiganavile Sridhar, G. Bartlett, et al. "Physicians' Assessment of the Value of Clinical Information: Operationalization of a Theoretical Model." *Journal of the Association for Information Science and Technology* 62, no. 10 (2011): 1884–91, doi:10.1002/asi.21590.

Grad, R., P. Pluye, J. Johnson-Lafleur, V. Granikov, M. Shulha, G. Bartlett, and B. Marlow. "Do Family Physicians Retrieve Synopses of Clinical Research Previously Read as Email Alerts?" *Journal of Medical Internet Research* 13, no. 4 (2011): e101, doi:10.2196/jmir.1683.

Grad, R.M., P. Pluye, C. Repchinsky, B. Jovaisas, B. Marlow, I.L.M. Ricarte, M.C.B. Galvão, M. Shulha, and J. de Gaspé Bonar. "Physician Assessments of the Value of Therapeutic Information Delivered via E-Mail." *Canadian Family Physician* 60, no. 5 (2014): e258-62.

Grad, R.M., P. Pluye, M. Shulha, D.L. Tang, J. Moscovici, C. Repchinsky, and J. Meuser. "Big Data from the Push of Clinical Information: Harvesting User Feedback for Continuing Education." In *Big Data and Health Analytics*, edited by K. Marconi and H. Lehmann, 79–103. Boca Raton, FL: CRC Press, Taylor & Francis, 2014.

Greenhalgh, T., E. Annandale, R. Ashcroft, J. Barlow, N. Black, A. Bleakley, R. Boaden, et al. "An Open Letter to the *BMJ* Editors on Qualitative Research." *British Medical Journal* 352 (2016): i563, doi:10.1136/bmj.i563.

Greenhalgh, T., J. Howick, and N. Maskrey. "Evidence Based Medicine: A Movement in Crisis?" *British Medical Journal* 348 (2014): g3725, doi:10.1136/bmj.g3725.

Gurteen, D. "Quotation from Sir Muir Gray." www.gurteen.com/gurteen/gurteen.nsf/id/knowledge-and-disease (accessed 27 November 2016).

Haggerty, J.L., R.J. Reid, G.K. Freeman, B.H. Starfield, C.E. Adair, and R. McKendry. "Continuity of Care: A Multidisciplinary Review." *British Medical Journal* 327, no. 7425 (2003): 1219–21, doi:10.1136/bmj.327.7425.1219.

Haynes, R.B., J. Holland, C. Cotoi, R.J. McKinlay, N.L. Wilczynski, L.A. Walters, D. Jedras, et al. "McMaster Plus: A Cluster

Randomized Clinical Trial of an Intervention to Accelerate Clinical Use of Evidence-Based Information from Digital Libraries." *Journal of the American Medical Informatics Association* 13, no. 6 (2006): 593–600, doi:10.1197/jamia.M2158.

Health Canada. "Canada Vigilance Adverse Reaction Online Database." Ottawa: Health Canada. www.hc-sc.gc.ca/dhp-mps/medeff/ databasdon/index-eng.php (accessed 27 November 2016).

Heath, I. "How Medicine Has Exploited Rationality at the Expense of Humanity: An Essay by Iona Heath." *British Medical Journal* 355 (2016): i5705, doi:10.1136/bmj.i5705.

Hersh, W.R. *Information Retrieval: A Health and Biomedical Perspective.* New York: Springer, 2009.

Hersh, W.R., M.K. Crabtree, D.H. Hickam, L. Sacherek, C.P. Friedman, P. Tidmarsh, C. Mosbaek, and D. Kraemer. "Factors Associated with Success in Searching MEDLINE and Applying Evidence to Answer Clinical Questions." *Journal of the American Medical Informatics Association* 9, no. 3 (2002): 283–93, doi:10.1197/ jamia.M0996.

Hersh, W.R., M.K. Crabtree, D.H. Hickam, L. Sacherek, L. Rose, and C.P. Friedman. "Factors Associated with Successful Answering of Clinical Questions Using an Information Retrieval System." *Bulletin of the Medical Library Association* 88, no. 4 (2000): 323–31.

Ioannidis, J.P. "Contradicted and Initially Stronger Effects in Highly Cited Clinical Research." *Journal of the American Medical Association* 294, no. 2 (2005): 218–28, doi:10.1001/jama.294.2.218.

Jorgenson, D., A. Muller, A.M. Whelan, and K. Buxton. "Pharmacists Teaching in Family Medicine Residency Programs National Survey." *Canadian Family Physician* 57, no. 9 (2011): e341–6.

Kahane, S., E. Stutz, and B. Aliarzadeh. "Must We Appear to Be All-Knowing?" *Canadian Family Physician* 57, no. 6 (2011): e228–36.

Kahneman, D. *Thinking Fast and Slow.* Toronto: Anchor Canada, 2011.

Knight, W. "AI's Language Problem." *MIT Technology Review* (9 August 2016). www.technologyreview.com/s/602094/ais-language-problem/

Labrecque, M., S. Ratté, P. Frémont, M. Cauchon, J. Ouellet, W. Hogg, J. McGowan, et al. "Decision Making in Family Medicine: Randomized Trial of the Effects of the Infoclinique and TRIP Database Search Engines." *Canadian Family Physician* 59, no. 10 (2013): 1084–94.

Landro, L. "With Chronic Care, Less Can Be More: Victor Montori at the Mayo Clinic Says That 'Minimally Disruptive Medicine' Can Lead to Better Health – and Lower Costs." *The Wall Street Journal*, 8 April 2013.

Lavoie, A., and C. Fontaine. "Mieux Connaître la Parentalité au Québec: Un Portrait à Partir de l'Enquête Québécoise sur l'Expérience des Parents d'Enfants de 0 à 5 Ans 2015." Québec, QC : Institut de la statistique du Québec, 2016. www.stat.gouv.qc.ca/statistiques/conditions-vie-societe/environnement-familial/eqepe.pdf (accessed 27 November 2016).

Légaré, F., S. Ratté, K. Gravel, and I.D. Graham. "Barriers and Facilitators to Implementing Shared Decision-Making in Clinical Practice: Update of a Systematic Review of Health Professionals' Perceptions." *Patient Education and Counseling* 73, no. 3 (2008): 526–35, doi:10.1016/j.pec.2008.07.018.

Légaré, F., D. Stacey, S. Gagnon, S. Dunn, P. Pluye, D. Frosch, J. Kryworuchko, et al. "Validating a Conceptual Model for an Interprofessional Approach to Shared Decision Making: A Mixed Methods Study." *Journal of Evaluation in Clinical Practice* 17, no. 4 (2011): 554–64, doi:10.1111/j.1365-2753.2010.01515.x.

Légaré, F., and H.O. Witteman. "Shared Decision Making: Examining Key Elements and Barriers to Adoption into Routine Clinical Practice." *Health Affairs (Millwood)* 32, no. 2 (2013): 276–84, doi:10.1377/hlthaff.2012.1078.

Liu, G.G., and D.B. Christensen. "The Continuing Challenge of Inappropriate Prescribing in the Elderly: An Update of the Evidence." *Journal of the American Pharmaceutical Association* 42, no. 6 (2002): 847–57, doi:10.1331/108658002762063682.

Luhmann, N. *Social Systems*. Stanford: Stanford University Press, 1995.

– "What Is Communication?" *Communication Theory* 2, no. 3 (1992): 251–9, doi:10.1111/j.1468-2885.1992.tb00042.x.

Malcolm, C.E., K.K. Wong, and R. Elwood-Martin. "Patients' Perceptions and Experiences of Family Medicine Residents in the Office." *Canadian Family Physician* 54, no. 4 (2008): 570–1.

McGaha, A.L., E. Garrett, A.C. Jobe, P. Nalin, W.P. Newton, P.A. Pugno, and N.B. Kahn Jr. "Responses to Medical Students' Frequently Asked Questions about Family Medicine." *American Family Physician* 76, no. 1 (2007): 99–106.

McKibbon, K.A., and D.B. Fridsma. "Effectiveness of Clinician-Selected Electronic Information Resources for Answering Primary Care Physicians' Information Needs." *Journal of the American Medical Informatics Association* 13, no. 6 (2006): 653–9, doi:10.1197/jamia.M2087.

McKibbon, K.A., C. Lokker, A. Keepanasseril, N.L. Wilczynski, and R.B. Haynes. "Net Improvement of Correct Answers to Therapy Questions after PubMed Searches: Pre/Post Comparison." *Journal of Medical Internet Research* 15, no. 11 (2013): e243, doi:10.2196/jmir.2572.

McNichol, B.R., and Rootman, I. "Literacy and Health Literacy: New Understandings about their Impact on Health." *Social Determinants of Health: Canadian Perspectives*, edited by D. Raphael, 261–90. Toronto: Canadian Scholars' Press; 2016.

Nahl, D. "Social–Biological Information Technology: An Integrated Conceptual Framework." *Journal of the Association for Information Science and Technology* 58, no. 13 (2007): 2021–46, doi:10.1002/asi.20690.

Nahl, D., and D. Bilal. *Information and Emotion: The Emergent Affective Paradigm in Information Behavior Research and Theory.* Medford, NJ: Information Today, 2007.

National Lung Screening Trial Research Team. "Reduced Lung-Cancer Mortality with Low-Dose Computed Tomographic Screening." *New England Journal of Medicine* 2011, no. 365 (2011): 395–409, doi:10.1056/NEJMoa1102873.

OCEBM Table of Evidence Working Group, J. Howick, I. Chalmers, P. Glasziou, T. Greenhalgh, A. Heneghan, I. Liberati, et al. "Oxford Centre for Evidence-Based Medicine 2011 Levels of Evidence." Oxford: Oxford Centre for Evidence-based Medicine, 2011. www.cebm.net/wp-content/uploads/2014/06/CEBM-Levels-of-Evidence-2.1.pdf (accessed 22 August 2016).

Organisation for Economic Co-operation and Development. "OECD Skills Outlook 2013: First Results from the Survey of Adult Skills [PIAAC Survey Volume 1]." Paris: OECD Publishing, 2013. http://dx.doi.org/10.1787/9789264204256-en (accessed 27 November 2016).

Pineault, R., R. Borges Da Silva, S. Provost, M.-D. Beaulieu, A. Boivin, A. Couture, and A. Prud'homme. "Primary Healthcare Solo Practices: Homogeneous or Heterogeneous?" *International Journal of Family Medicine* 2014 (2014): 1–10, doi:10.1155/2014/373725.

Pluye, P., R.M. Grad, L.G. Dunikowski, and R. Stephenson. "Impact of Clinical Information-Retrieval Technology on Physicians: A Literature Review of Quantitative, Qualitative and Mixed Methods Studies." *International Journal of Medical Informatics* 74, no. 9 (2005): 745–68, doi:10.1016/j.ijmedinf.2005.05.004.

Pluye, P., R.M. Grad, J. Johnson-Lafleur, V. Granikov, M. Shulha, B. Marlow, and I. Ricarte. "The Number Needed to Benefit from Information (NNBI): Proposal from a Mixed Methods Research Study with Practicing Family Physicians." *Annals of Family Medicine* 11, no. 6 (2013): 559–67, doi:10.1370/afm.1565.

Pluye, P., R.M. Grad, N. Mysore, L. Knaapen, J. Johnson-Lafleur, and M. Dawes. "Systematically Assessing the Situational Relevance of Electronic Knowledge Resources: A Mixed Methods Study." *Journal of the American Medical Informatics Association* 14, no. 5 (2007): 616–25, doi:10.1197/jamia.M2203.

Pluye, P., R.M. Grad, N. Mysore, M. Shulha, and J. Johnson-Lafleur. "Using Electronic Knowledge Resources for Person Centered Medicine - Part 2: The Number Needed to Benefit from Information (NNBI)." *International Journal of Person Centered Medicine* 1, no. 2 (2011b): 395–404, doi:10.5750/ijpcm.v1i2.83.

Pluye, P., R.M. Grad, C. Repchinsky, B. Farrell, J. Johnson-Lafleur, T. Bambrick, M. Dawes, et al. "IAM: A Comprehensive and Systematic Information Assessment Method for Electronic Knowledge Resources." In *Handbook of Research on Information Technology Management and Clinical Data Administration in Healthcare*, edited by A. Dwivedi, 521–48. Hershey, PA: IGI Publishing, 2009.

Pluye, P., R.M. Grad, C. Repchinsky, B. Jovaisas, J. Johnson-Lafleur, M.E. Carrier, V. Granikov, et al. "Four Levels of Outcomes of Information-Seeking: A Mixed Methods Study in Primary Health Care." *Journal of the Association for Information Science and Technology* 64, no. 1 (2013): 108–25, doi:10.1002/asi.22793.

Pluye, P., R.M. Grad, M. Shulha, V. Granikov, and K. Leung. "Using Electronic Knowledge Resources for Person Centered Medicine – Part 1: An Evaluation Model." *International Journal of Person Centered Medicine* 1, no. 2 (2011a): 385–94, doi:10.5750/ijpcm.v1i2.82.

Pluye, P., V. Granikov, G. Bartlett, R.M. Grad, D.L. Tang, J. Johnson-Lafleur, M. Shulha, et al. "Development and Content Validation of the Information Assessment Method for Patients and Consumers." *Journal of Medical Internet Research Research Protocols* 3, no. 1 (2014): e7, doi:10.2196/resprot.2908.

Pluye, P., and Q.N. Hong. "Combining the Power of Stories and the Power of Numbers: Mixed Methods Research and Mixed Studies Reviews." *Annual Review of Public Health* 35 (2014): 29–45, doi: 10.1146/annurev-publhealth-032013-182440.

Pluye, P., R.E. Sherif, G. Bartlett, V. Granikov, R.M. Grad, G. Doray, F. Lagarde, C. Loignon, and F. Bouthillier. "Perceived Outcomes of Online Parenting Information According to Self-Selected Participants from a Population of Website Users." *Proceedings of the Association for Information Science and Technology* 52, no. 1 (2015): 1–3, doi:10.1002/pra2.2015.145052010072.

Radley, D.C., S.N. Finkelstein, and R.S. Stafford. "Off-Label Prescribing among Office-Based Physicians." *Archives of Internal Medicine* 166, no. 9 (2006): 1021–6, doi:10.1001/archinte.166.9.1021.

Roger, V.L., A.S. Go, D.M. Lloyd-Jones, E.J. Benjamin, J.D. Berry, W.B. Borden, D.M. Bravata, et al. "Heart Disease and Stroke Statistics – 2012 Update. A Report from the American Heart

Association." *Circulation* 125, no. 1 (2012): e2–220, doi:10.1161/CIR.0b013e31823ac046.

Roots, A., and M. MacDonald. "Outcomes Associated with Nurse Practitioners in Collaborative Practice with General Practitioners in Rural Settings in Canada: A Mixed Methods Study." *Human Resources for Health* 12 (2014): 69, doi:10.1186/1478-4491-12-69.

Rouleau, G., M.-P. Gagnon, and J. Côté. "Impacts of Information and Communication Technologies on Nursing Care: An Overview of Systematic Reviews (Protocol)." *Systematic Reviews* 4, (2015): 75, doi:10.1186/s13643-015-0062-y.

Sackett, D.L., W.M.C. Rosenberg, J.A.M. Gray, R.B. Haynes, and W.S. Richardson. "Evidence-Based Medicine: What It Is and What It Is Not." *British Medical Journal* 312, no. 7023 (1996): 71–2, doi:10.1136/bmj.312.7023.71.

Saracevic, T., and P.B. Kantor. "Studying the Value of Library and Information Services. Part I. Establishing a Theoretical Framework." *Journal of the Association for Information Science and Technology* 48, no. 6 (1997): 527–42, doi:10.1002/(SICI)1097-4571(199706)48:6<527::AID-ASI6>3.0.CO;2-w.

Siegel, E.R., R.A. Logan, R.L. Harnsberger, K. Cravedi, J.A. Krause, B. Lyon, K. Hajarian, et al. "Information Rx: Evaluation of a New Informatics Tool for Physicians, Patients, and Libraries." *Information Services and Use* 26, no. 1 (2006): 1–10, doi:10.1080/15398280902896493.

Siegel, R.L., K.D. Miller, and A. Jemal. "Cancer Statistics, 2015." CA: *A Cancer Journal for Clinicians* 65, no. 1 (2015): 5–29, doi:10.3322/caac.21254.

Simon, H.A. *The Sciences of the Artificial.* Cambridge, MA: MIT Press, 1969.

Slawson, D.C. "Teaching Evidence-Based Medicine: Should We Be Teaching Information Management Instead?" [Oral Presentation]. www.youtube.com/watch?v=w6oYNt3deW4 (accessed 27 November 2016).

Slawson, D.C., and A.F. Shaughnessy. "Teaching Evidence-Based Medicine: Should We Be Teaching Information Management Instead?" *Academic Medicine* 80, no. 7 (2005): 685–9.

Slawson, D.C., A. F. Shaughnessy, and J. H. Bennett. "Becoming a Medical Information Master: Feeling Good about Not Knowing Everything." *Journal of Family Practice* 38, no. 5 (1994): 505–13.

Statistics Canada. "Canadian Internet Use Survey." Ottawa: Statistics Canada, 2010. www.statcan.gc.ca/daily-quotidien/110525/dq110525b-eng.htm (accessed 27 November 2016).

– "Health State Descriptions for Canadians: Mental Illnesses – Section C: Childhood Conditions." Ottawa: Statistics Canada. www.statcan.gc.ca/pub/82-619-m/2012004/sections/sectionc-eng.htm (accessed 27 November 2016).

Stern, D.T. "A Framework for Measuring Medical Professionalism." In *Measuring Medical Professionalism*, edited by D.T. Stern, 3–13. New York: Oxford University Press, 2006.

Sullivan, F.M., and R.J. MacNaughton. "Evidence in Consultations: Interpreted and Individualised." *The Lancet* 348, no. 9032 (1996): 941–3, doi:10.1016/S0140-6736(96)05219-1.

Tamblyn, R., A. Huang, R. Perreault, A. Jacques, D. Roy, J. Hanley, P. McLeod, and R. Laprise. "The Medical Office of the 21st Century (MOXXI): Effectiveness of Computerized Decision-Making Support in Reducing Inappropriate Prescribing in Primary Care." *Canadian Medical Aassociation Journal* 169, no. 6 (2003): 549–56.

Tonsaker, T., G. Bartlett, and C. Trpkov. "Health Information on the Internet: Gold Mine or Minefield?" *Canadian Family Physician* 60, no. 5 (2014): 407–8.

Tu, H.T., and G.R. Cohen. "Striking Jump in Consumers Seeking Health Care Information." *Tracking Report – Center for Studying Health System Change* no. 20 (2008): 1–8.

Veroff, D., A. Marr, and D.E. Wennberg. "Enhanced Support for Shared Decision Making Reduced Costs of Care for Patients with Preference-Sensitive Conditions." *Health Affairs (Millwood)* 32, no. 2 (2013): 285–93, doi:10.1377/hlthaff.2011.0941.

Weiss, B.D., and J.G. Schwartzberg. *Health Literacy and Patient Safety: Help Patients Understand. Manual for Clinicians*. Chicago: American Medical Association Foundation, 2007.

Welch, H.G. "Overdiagnosed: Making People Sick in the Pursuit of Health." [Oral Presentation]. www.youtube.com/watch?v=6NbRp A7yeMI (accessed 27 November 2016).

Wellbery, C., and R.A. McAteer. "When Medicine Reverses Itself: Avoiding Practice Pitfalls." *American Family Physician* 88 (2013): 733–8.

Westbrook, J.I., E.W. Coiera, and A.S. Gosling. "Do Online Information Retrieval Systems Help Experienced Clinicians Answer Clinical Questions?" *Journal of the American Medical Informatics Association* 12, no. 3 (2005): 315–21, doi:10.1197/jamia.M1717.

Westbrook, J.I., E.W. Coiera, A.S. Gosling, and J. Braithwaite. "Critical Incidents and Journey Mapping as Techniques to Evaluate the Impact of Online Evidence Retrieval Systems on Health Care Delivery and Patient Outcomes." *International Journal of Medical Informatics* 76, no. 2–3 (2007): 234–45, doi:10.1016/j.ijmedinf. 2006.03.006.

White, B. "Making Evidence-Based Medicine Doable in Everyday Practice." *Family Practice Management* 11, no. 2 (2004): 51–8.

White, R.W., and E. Horvitz. "Experiences with Web Search on Medical Concerns and Self-Diagnosis." *American Medical Informatics Association Annual Symposium Proceedings* 2009 (2009): 696–700.

– "Cyberchondria: Studies of the Escalation of Medical Concerns in Web Search." ACM *Transactions on Information Systems* 27, no. 4 (2009): 1–37.

Winterstein, A.G., S. Linden, A.E. Lee, E.M. Fernandez, and C.L. Kimberlin. "Evaluation of Consumer Medication Information Dispensed in Retail Pharmacies." *Archives of Internal Medicine* 170, no. 15 (2010): 1317–24, doi:10.1001/archinternmed.2010.263.

Ylinen, J., E.-P. Takala, M. Nykänen, A. Häkkinen, E. Mälkiä, T. Pohjolainen, S.-L. Karppi, H. Kautiainen, and O. Airaksinen. "Active Neck Muscle Training in the Treatment of Chronic Neck Pain in Women: A Randomized Controlled Trial." *Journal of the American Medical Association* 289, no. 19 (2003): 2509–16, doi:10.1001/jama.289.19.2509.

Index